The Yin & Yang of Cancer

BREAKTHROUGHS FROM
THE EAST AND THE WEST

Bernard Chan, M.D.
Georges M. Halpern, M.D., Ph.D.

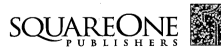
SQUAREONE
PUBLISHERS

The information and advice in this book are based on the training, personal experiences, and research of the author. Its contents are current and accurate; however, the information presented is not intended to substitute for professional medical advice. The author and the publisher urge you to consult with your physician or other qualified health-care provider prior to starting any treatment or undergoing any surgical procedure. Because there is always some risk involved, the author and publisher cannot be responsible for any adverse effects or consequences resulting from the use of any of the suggestions, preparations, or procedures described in this book.

COVER DESIGNER: Jeannie Tudor
EDITOR: John Anderson
TYPESETTER: Gary A. Rosenberg

Square One Publishers
115 Herricks Road
Garden City Park, NY 11040
(516) 535-2010 • (877) 900-BOOK
www.squareonepublishers.com

Library of Congress Cataloging-in-Publication Data

Chan, Bernard, 1935-
  The yin and yang of cancer : breakthroughs from East and West /
Bernard Chan and Georges Halpern.
      p. ; cm.
  Includes bibliographical references and index.
  ISBN-13: 978-0-7570-0207-6 (quality pbk.)
  ISBN-10: 0-7570-0207-2 (quality pbk.)
  1. Cancer—Treatment. 2. Medicine, Chinese. 3. Integrative medicine. I.
Halpern, Georges M. II. Title.
  [DNLM: 1. Neoplasms—therapy. 2. Agaricales. 3. Cross-Cultural Comparison.
4. Medicine, Chinese Traditional. 5. Phytotherapy. QZ 266 C454y 2007]

RC270.8.C42 2007
616.99'4—dc22
                              2007025446

Printed in the United States of America

10   9   8   7   6   5   4   3   2   1

Contents

Acknowledgments

We have been inspired by the many cancer patients who taught us lessons in humanity and grace. Without them, we could not have written this book.

We thank Rudy Shur, our publisher, who accepted our book to his prestigious catalog; John Anderson, our editor; Peter Weverka, Andrew Miller, and John Holliday, who contributed ideas to various chapters; other mentors, colleagues, and friends at the many institutions, both in the East and in the West, where we have worked.

Finally, our work is dedicated to our wives, Dieneke and Emiko, who have been unfailingly patient and understanding.

Bernard Chan
Georges Halpern

Introduction

This book is about cancer, a great modern plague, but it is about much more. Its broader themes, touched on throughout, include how science and medicine evolve and how different cultures in medicine interact with and change one another. It is about the great advances we have made in understanding cancer, but it is also about the tragedy of the millions still dying of this dreaded disease every year. It is also a scientific look at the use of medicinal mushrooms, which the Chinese have used for centuries to treat cancer.

In science and medicine, problems sometimes remain unsolved for decades, even centuries, engendering controversies beyond their fields—to ethics, to morality, and to society at large. Yet, when they are finally solved, there may be no "Eureka!" moment: the transition from the past way of thinking to the present way of thinking may be so seamless, and the new way so natural, that we wonder why there was any fuss at all. Thomas Kuhn, who popularized the term *paradigm,* called these transitions "invisible revolutions." In his book *The Structure of Scientific Revolutions,* Kuhn, one of the most influential thinkers of the twentieth century, argues that scientific progress may be seen as a series of crises and responses to crises, which are part of the nature and necessity of science. His central theme is that scientists cling to an old and dysfunctional paradigm, modifying it as they go along, until a new paradigm is ready. This is especially true where an advance involves a new worldview.

Historically, one of the most famous "paradigm shifts" was associated with the discovery of Galileo Galilei (1564–1642) that the Earth revolves around the sun and not vice versa, as the church authorities and most philosophers of Galileo's time insisted. This was not, as Kuhn pointed out, an abrupt change in astronomical science, coming as it were out of a clear blue sky. Rather, it evolved as the older model of the sun revolving around the Earth became increasingly untenable. Many modifications of the old model were tried and each modification appeared workable for a while. Interestingly, Kuhn pointed out that scientists (and in those days, there was no distinction between science and philosophy) persisted in the cumbersome old model with its many, sometimes contradictory, modifications, until a new paradigm was ready. Nowadays, we often think of the Galileo story as an abrupt event, since the Inquisition threatened to torture him until he recanted. Thus, he became a hero of the scientific Enlightenment and a big stick that some scientists (but not all) still use to hit back at the church. But this has nothing to do with the paradigm shift, which is nearly always an invisible revolution, and more to do with a peculiar attitude, which may be called "fundamentalism."

A GREAT MODERN PLAGUE

Cancer kills more than four million people each year. Many people are newly diagnosed with some form of cancer each year, and nearly everyone knows someone, a close friend or relative, with cancer. The book is written for them, the cancer sufferers and their families, as well as the dedicated professionals who care for them. This book will trace the history of cancer medicine from ancient times to the present, and look at the very considerable progress in Western medicine, but without an attitude of fundamentalism.

From the standpoint of mainstream medicine, there is both good news and bad news regarding cancer. The good news is that some treatments are working—many forms of childhood cancer can be cured with present day treatments. The bad news is that, for the majority of advanced cancers, conventional treatment doesn't work very well. That is why there is, we believe, an ongoing invisible revolution in the way we think about cancer, both from the scientific and medical standpoint and from that of the lay public, including the millions of cancer sufferers.

A paradigm is more than theory alone but less than the sum of all relevant theories and practice. It involves frameworks, shared rules, and what might be called "normal" science. In cancer medicine, as in astronomy, it is the everyday practice of normal science exposing contradictions between theory and practice that drives forward the invisible revolution. For example, in the 1960s and 1970s, it was found that chemotherapy could cure some cases of childhood leukemia and that more chemotherapy—stronger doses and combinations of drugs—could cure more cases of leukemia, including even some adults with the disease. Doctors then proceeded to treat many cancers with strong chemotherapy, but with meager results. In retrospect, they might have fallen for the "black raven fallacy": if it is true that all ravens are black, then it logically follows that all non-black objects are not ravens; but it is a fallacy to think that all black objects are ravens.

COMPLEMENTARY AND ALTERNATIVE MEDICINE FOR CANCER

There is another aspect to the story. Cancer sufferers are increasingly interested in "integrative medicine," a newly emerging field in which complementary and alternative methods of healing are combined with mainstream Western medicine. In many ways, this represents a cry from the heart, a tremor of existential anguish for medicine to hear. What is complementary and alternative medicine (CAM)? It has been defined as a group of diverse medical and health-care systems, practices, and products that are not presently considered to be part of conventional medicine. While scientific evidence exists regarding some CAM therapies, there are key questions that are yet to be answered through well-designed scientific studies, such as whether such therapies are safe and if they work for the diseases or medical conditions for which they are used. Cancer patients have one of the highest rates of CAM use—it is estimated that up to 83 percent of cancer patients use some form of CAM at some point.

In the past fifteen years, CAM practices have gained the attention and interest of many academic institutions. The Society for Integrative Oncology has recently been founded as an international organization for oncology professionals to promote the interaction between mainstream cancer medicine and CAM. What is meant by "integrative oncology," both in theory and in practice? One way to answer that question is to look at the use of Chinese medicine for cancer, which has a 5,000-year tradition and which forms a large component of CAM. The People's Republic of China, the world's most populous nation, has a very high rate of utilization of CAM. This book will look, albeit only briefly, at how integrative medicine works in China and discuss whether there are lessons from the Chinese experience in integrative oncology for the West. A detailed discussion of medicinal mushrooms is included, since they are the main ingredients in herbal treatments for cancer.

FROM OPPOSITE ENDS OF THE EARTH

About two years before the end of the Second World War, the authors discovered the joys of mushrooms, but it was much later that we came to understand their medicinal properties. We were children then, growing up on opposite ends of the earth. There were few toys, and like children almost everywhere, we loved to explore our natural surroundings. We knew every nook in the neighborhood, every tree in the nearby woods where we would go after school. And, of course, school was often interrupted by the war, and so those exploratory trips to the woods often took the place of school.

We knew the small animals and birds that we would find in the woods. We could recognize the fragrance of the fields in different seasons, and after summer rains, we would often find mushrooms in the woods. We were two young boys, the one living in a refugee camp in Switzerland and the other on a farm in southern China, which was at that time occupied by the Japanese Imperial Army. Our parents did not discourage us from looking for mushrooms but told us that some were poisonous and some were edible, indeed delicious. Both of us went on to study medicine after the war and became interested in the treatment of cancer. We both retained our fascination with mushrooms, both as a culinary delicacy and as we gradually became aware of their legendary healing properties.

We did not meet until much later. Georges studied in Paris, practiced as a doctor, first in France and then he later emigrated to the United States, where he became a professor in internal medicine, nutrition, and pharmacology. His interests led him to conduct research in the rapidly expanding sciences of molecular medicine. Still later, he studied the active ingredients in herbal medicine, particularly traditional Chinese medicine. Something within has always drawn him toward the East, and after more than twenty years of teaching in California, he went to Hong Kong and became a distinguished professor in pharmaceutical sciences.

Bernard went in the opposite direction. Whereas Georges, the young boy from the refugee camp in Switzerland, became interested in China, Bernard, the young Chinese boy, went to the West. He studied in London and Cambridge and became a doctor, first in England and then in Canada. His field was hematology and his interests led him to study bone marrow transplantation and cellular therapy for cancer.

We eventually met and found that we had many things in common, one of which was an interest in medicinal mushrooms. Out of our friendship came this book.

THE JOURNEY AHEAD

The plan for this book is simple: alternate chapters are written from a Western and from an Eastern standpoint. By a curious twist of fate, Bernard, originally from China, will contribute the Western perspective. This includes a chapter on the history of cancer treatment from ancient times to the modern development of surgery, radiation oncology, and chemotherapy. He also tells the story of bone marrow transplantation, an undoubted triumph of scientific medicine. A chapter called "The Dark Valley" describes how, despite vast resources over many decades, suffering and death still await the majority of people found to have cancer. "New Beginnings" discusses recent developments of molecular targeted therapy and cell therapy, and the story of cancer vaccines and immunotherapy is covered in another chapter.

Georges, with extensive research interest in medicinal mushrooms, is responsible for the Eastern perspective, although there was much cross-fertilization of ideas. Alternative views of disease in different cultures are discussed—for example, the Chinese concept of disease as a lack of balance in the body rather than simply a failure in a mechanical system, the predominant idea in Western medicine. The cultural and philosophical basis for the practice of medicine in China is described briefly. "A Visit to a Chinese Hospital" takes the reader on a tour to the world of integrative medicine in China, where Western medicine and traditional Chinese medicine are truly partners. Another chapter tells the story of how herbs came to be used for healing, including the story of culinary mushrooms that also have significant medicinal properties. This is followed by a discussion of *lingzhi* and *yunzhi,* two mushrooms commonly used to treat cancer in China, as well as the fabled story of a healing mushroom that also has an amazing life cycle inside an insect.

But in what sense is the use of mushrooms a breakthrough? After all, mushrooms have been around since before civilization and their use as rare and precious herbs for Chinese emperors has been documented for hundreds of years. The answer lies in the more recent domestication of mushrooms and the manufacture of their products on an industrial scale. Medicinal mushrooms offered to the emperors were rare specimens collected from the wild—now they are available to all of us.

The book closes with a chapter entitled "The Quest for Common Ground," in which we look at how both East and West can share a common approach focused on utilizing the immune system to fight cancer, and we discuss cultural and other barriers that need to be overcome before a full partnership can be realized.

1

Times of Hope

CANCER IN THE ANCIENT WORLD

Cancer was well known in the ancient world. In Greece, one of the earliest records of the disease appeared in *Papyrus* in approximately 1600 BC, but it may have been based on even earlier writings, perhaps dating back as far as 3000 BC. Hippocrates (c. 460–377 BC) and Galen (c. AD 129–199) knew about the "crab-like" (the meaning of the word *karkinos* in Greek) disease that grew uncontrollably, ultimately killing the victim. One of Hippocrates' aphorisms was on the treatment of hiccups, a common symptom of cancer of the upper digestive tract: "In the case of a person afflicted with hiccough, sneezing coming on removes the hiccough." This remains a true observation and is still quoted in modern textbooks.

Studies of Egyptian mummies provide a fascinating glimpse, including diseases and medical procedures, into the ancient world. These showed evidence of different types of cancer, including those of the female reproductive organs and of the digestive tract, and even of surgical procedures carried out apparently with curative intent. Herbs were used to treat cancer in several ancient cultures, including China and Tibet, with extensive descriptions of different combinations and their indications passed down through oral traditions and written texts.

There was not yet a science of pathology in the modern sense and methods of diagnosis were rudimentary. Most of the surgery carried out in those early times was the removal of superficial tumors, although there was at least one report of an operation to remove a brain tumor in ancient China. Even then, the goal of the surgeon was to operate electively, with a minimum of pain and to achieve a high rate of success. This was particularly important since the patient was frequently a high official or a member of the aristocracy, and sometimes the king or emperor himself—dire consequences would result for unlucky surgical operators. Even in the modern era, cancer surgery retains its position as the mode of therapy that achieves the highest rates of cure.

THE BEGINNING OF THE MODERN ERA

It took many centuries and a number of critical developments in science and technology before cancer treatment gained public acceptance. Surgery continued to play a pivotal role, not only as a bedside science but also in the organization and reform of hospitals. Many achievements by surgical pioneers, particularly in the United Kingdom and United States in the eighteenth and nineteenth centuries, survive to the present day. These include improvements in sanitation and ventilation, as well as the provision of less crowded hospital rooms, all of which tended to reduce the rate of infections.

The first reported elective surgery in modern times was the removal of a gigantic ovarian tumor by Ephraim McDowell in 1809. The tumor weighed twenty-two pounds and the patient survived to live another thirty years. This amazing accomplishment was before the era of antisepsis and anesthesia. With the development of these important innovations, cancer surgery rapidly progressed. Today, many surgical procedures are performed using minimally invasive techniques, so-called "keyhole" surgery, and cancer surgeons are integrated into a multidisciplinary team.

Medical discoveries often occur as the result of a lucky break and sometimes of unusual circumstances. This was true of the earliest application of anesthesia, which was associated with Crawford Long, a dentist who had a large practice in the state of Georgia in the 1840s. This successful and gregarious doctor often entertained his friends in his opulently furnished home. Although conservatively dressed, with a grayish beard and of a solemn demeanor, he was at heart something of a hippie and would invite his friends to his home for "ether parties." Sniffing ether would enable the good doctor and his companions to enjoy a temporary loss of southern inhibitions, a practice which would horrify his present day professional colleagues, not to mention invite the interest of law enforcement. However, he did make the important discovery that not only did his friends lose their inhibitions, they also lost their sense of pain as well.

In 1846, John Warren carried out the first recorded cancer surgery using ether anesthesia. This was the removal of a tongue cancer from a patient named Gilbert Abbott. Another dentist, William Morton, who personally developed the technique based on Long's observations, administered the ether and so became the first medical specialist of anesthesia.

ASEPTIC SURGICAL TECHNIQUES

The birth of modern surgery is usually associated with the name Joseph Lister. Lister was the son of a successful Quaker wine merchant who was also an accomplished inventor, having designed the first modern achromatic microscope. In 1846, Lister was an art student in London when, quite by chance, he was a spectator at the first surgical operation using general anesthesia to be performed in England. The experience made a great impression on Lister and he decided to study medicine, qualifying as a surgeon in 1852 and working first in Edinburgh and Glasgow, then later in London.

At that time, surgery was frequently followed by infection or "putrefaction" as it was then called. The role of microorganisms in the process of inflammation was not yet understood, with Louis Pasteur (1822–1895) just beginning his epoch-making studies of "fermentation" in 1857, which would lead him to develop the germ theory of disease. In 1846, Ignaz Semmelweis, a Hungarian physician in Vienna, had shown that sepsis, particularly following childbirth in the hospital, could be dramatically reduced when surgeons washed their hands. His findings, however, were ignored.

At the hospitals where Lister worked, the mortality rate from amputation surgery was as high as 50 percent, with almost all deaths due to infection. Abdominal surgery carried even greater risks. Such operations were rarely performed and then only by the brave or the reckless. Lister had read the work published by Pasteur and understood the similarity between sepsis and the fermentation described in Pasteur's experiments. By this time, Lister himself was an accomplished surgeon, and introduced the use of the antiseptic carbolic acid to kill bacteria in the operating rooms. This was dramatically successful in reducing postoperative infections. His methods were quickly adopted in Germany, especially during the Franco-Prussian War of 1870, with astonishing results on the battlefield.

Lister made numerous other innovations, such as the use of absorbable ligatures and the drainage tube. His senior colleagues in England did not always appreciate his innovations, although they were quickly adopted, not only on the continent but also across the Atlantic. The further development of aseptic techniques (preventing bacteria from entering the operative field) soon revolutionized surgery, especially in relation to cancer.

DISCOVERING THE CELLULAR AND MOLECULAR BASIS OF CANCER

In 1621, the microscope was invented, so laying the foundation of modern cellular science. The early microscopes were very crude and usually consisted of a single lens. Progress was slow, as there was no clear concept as to what was being revealed by this new instrument. The noted Italian biologist Marcello Malphigi was born in 1628, the year in which William Harvey published his celebrated paper *"De motu cordis"* heralding a new era of anatomy and physiology. Malphigi graduated in philosophy from the University of Bologna and then turned to medicine, becoming a doctor in 1653. His work on microscopy became well known throughout continental Europe and was also published by the Royal Society in London. Working with a frog lung, he discovered capillary circulation. The frog was a fortuitous choice, as its lungs are almost transparent and could be studied using single-lens microscopic techniques, but we had to wait almost two centuries before the next significant steps.

In the nineteenth century, the German pathologist Rudolf Virchow (1821–1902) formulated his theory of the cellular basis of cancer, laying the foundations of the modern understanding of the disease. He recognized leukemia in 1845 and went on to study the cellular basis of other blood diseases and parasites. During the final decades of the nineteenth century and the beginning of the twentieth, the discoveries of Marie Curie, Konrad Roentgen, Theodor Boveri, Paul Ehrlich, and others ushered in the modern era of cancer medicine as a science of cellular pathology. These innovators were truly modern ("modernity" itself being a modern invention) and developed the naturalistic view of illness, as something having natural causes and amenable to treatment by removal of these causes. They represented a total break with the classical tradition of medicine as a study to rediscover the works of Hippocrates, Galen, and Aristotle.

Today, few people outside a small academic circle know the name of the German geneticist Theodor Boveri (1862–1915), although he was highly regarded during his lifetime. One of his contem-poraries, E.B. Wilson, who was himself a well-known developmental biologist, wrote: "Boveri stood without a rival among biologists of his generation, and his writings will long endure as classical models."

Boveri began as a student of history and philosophy at the University of Munich, in Germany. He soon recognized the importance of deductive principles in philosophy, which was becoming increasingly "scientific." After graduating in medicine, he taught anatomy for a time at Munich and Würzburg. Like most biologists of his time, he based his studies on simple organisms, in this case, sea urchins' eggs. Work on the fertilization of sea urchins' eggs by two instead of one sperm showed that distribution of unequal numbers of chromosomes to the daughter cells led to specific characteristics, depending on the random combination of the chromosomes. From this work, he developed the chromosomal theory of heredity.

All living creatures begin life as single cells that divide and whose progeny continually divide according to a unique set of coded instructions in the DNA (deoxyribonucleic acid) of the cell nucleus. The parts of this code, each defining a specific function, are called genes. There are approximately 100,000 genes in the nucleus of a mammalian cell. Chromosomes are strings of genes. During the process of cell division, each chromosome has to be duplicated and one copy of each is passed on to the daughter cells. Human beings have 23 pairs of chromosomes in each cell, including a pair of so-called sex chromosomes; in the female, both sex chromosomes are X chromosomes, whereas in the male there is one X and one Y chromosome.

Boveri made the connection between the abnormal growth of sea urchins' eggs that carried the "wrong" chromosomes and the growth of malignant tumors. In 1914, he published the celebrated *Zur Frage der Entstehung Maligner Tumoren* (*The Origin of Malignant Tumors*). The term *gene* had not yet been invented in Boveri's time, but if we insert the word "gene" where Boveri had "chromosomes" in his thesis (after all chromosomes are long strings of genes), we have the modern version of the cellular basis of cancer genetics.

Boveri was exceptionally prophetic, stating that "in every normal cell there is a specific arrangement for inhibiting, which allows the process of division to begin only when the inhibition has been overcome by a specific stimulus. To assume the presence of definite chromosomes, which inhibits division, would harmonize best with my fundamental idea . . . cells of tumors with unlimited growth would arise if those inhibiting chromosomes were eliminated." He had, in that passage, correctly described the concepts of oncogenes and tumor suppressor genes, two important principles of the molecular basis of cancer.

Modern science has identified particular genes in normal DNA that direct the production of growth factors, which are like cellular hormones communicating between different cells, controlling the process of growth. When such genes are components of processes that may lead to abnormal growth or cancer, they are called proto-oncogenes. These do not themselves cause cancer, and indeed they are part of the genetic makeup of all healthy individuals. Only when mutations occur, such as due to a break-up of a chromosome at that particular point or when mistakes occur when pieces of chromosomes are incorrectly joined together, can these protooncogenes turn into oncogenes, causing cancer. Even so, it generally takes several steps for the process to become cancerous. Tumor suppressor genes work in the opposite direction and, only if they are accidentally turned off during a breakup or rearrangement of chromosomes, does the process lead to malignancy.

Boveri was so ahead of his time that the next significant discovery would not occur until 1960—the discovery of the "Philadelphia chromosome," a mutation that joins together pieces of different chromosomes, leading to the activation of cellular genetic mechanisms that cause some types of leukemia. In modern practice, the analysis of chromosomes in the cells of leukemia and some other types of cancer has become a routine part of diagnosis, allowing physicians to determine whether a particular cancer belongs to a high- or low-risk category and to design treatment accordingly. This scientific method, called cytogenetics, has evolved from the original technique of analysis of chromosomes in dividing cells to include the use of fluorescent probes of DNA in non-dividing cells and the direct analysis of DNA fragments. For example, thousands of fragments of DNA from tumors can be sprayed onto slides and analyzed by computer and the results used to determine treatment and prognosis. This modern advance, called microarrays, is a direct result of Boveri's predictions.

X-RAYS AND RADIOLOGY

Today, we take for granted the radiologist's capability to see inside the body using invisible rays to create an image of internal organs. However, the discovery of x-rays came quite by chance in 1895 to Konrad Roentgen, who was a professor of physics at the University of Würzburg, in Germany, when he made his famous discovery. Like many other scientists of that time, he was experimenting with cathode ray tubes through which an electric current was passed. Since the tube glowed brightly, he wondered if some rays were escaping that he could not detect with the naked eye because the fluorescence was so bright. He covered the tube in light-opaque material and darkened the room, the better to view the rays, which he imagined to be dim. By coincidence, there was a plate covered with fluorescent material lying on the bench and it glowed brightly even though no rays were visible in the intervening space. He called these "x-rays." In one experiment, he interposed his wife's hand between the cathode tube and a photographic plate—the result was the world's first x-ray picture.

The publication of Roentgen's discovery caused a sensation, and within a year more than forty laboratories were experimenting with x-rays. Roentgen was awarded the first Nobel Prize for physics in 1901 "for the discovery of the remarkable rays subsequently named after him." However, he was a modest man and discouraged the use of the term *Roentgen rays*, preferring the simpler name x-rays. To his considerable credit, he resisted the temptation to patent his discovery, thus allowing the new science of radiology to rapidly develop. He died in poverty during the hyperinflation of the Weimar Republic in Germany following the First World War.

Roentgen's discovery led directly to today's sophisticated diagnostic imaging technology, including very high speed computer-assisted tomography (CT) scans and magnetic resonance imaging (MRI), both of which can give accurate three-dimensional images with great detail. More recently, positron emission tomography (PET) scans, which utilize isotopes actively metabolized by tumor cells, combine detection of tumors with assessment of their activity.

RADIATION THERAPY

Perhaps the greatest pioneer of that era was Marie Curie, born Manya Sklodowska. Poland, where she grew up, was strongly dominated by Russia at that time. Her father was a teacher of mathematics and physics and her mother the principal of a girls' school. As a teenager, she was fascinated by science, but the family was poor and there were no science high schools for girls in Poland. Manya took a post as a governess and helped her sister Bronya to become a doctor in Paris. After qualifying in medicine, it was Bronya's turn to help Manya. In 1891, Manya went to Paris to study physics and proved to be a brilliant student and a perfectionist, at the top of her class at the Sorbonne. After graduation, she met Pierre Curie, then 35 years old and working at the Industrial School of Physics and Chemistry. Manya put off her plans to return to Poland and the two were married.

In addition to Konrad Roentgen, a number of other scientists in the 1890s were also fascinated by the phenomenon of fluorescence. Several researchers speculated that fluorescent substances were also capable of giving out the newly described x-rays. However, fluorescence was also thought to be in response to exposure to bright light. Henri Becquerel, a French physicist, decided to investigate the relationship between light exposure and fluorescence. He wrapped a photographic plate in lightproof paper, together with some uranium salts, and exposed the combination to bright sunlight. He found that the photographic plate contained a picture of the uranium crystals when it was developed. When he tried to repeat the experiment, the weather was cloudy and he did not make the exposure. The matter was forgotten until some weeks later when the unexposed plate was developed. Much to Becquerel's surprise, the plate also contained a picture of the uranium crystals—sunlight was therefore unnecessary.

Becquerel was fascinated. He suggested that his friend Pierre Curie's brilliant young wife should investigate the phenomenon. Marie took to it immediately and was soon joined by Pierre. One of the first materials they studied was the mineral pitchblende, which is approximately 60 percent uranium. However, the radioactivity (the name Marie gave to the mysterious new rays) of pitchblende was higher than that of pure uranium. The Curies concluded that the ore must contain other material with higher radioactivity. Soon, through numerous chemical analyses and purifications, they discovered a new element, which Marie named polonium in honor of her native country. A few months later, they discovered a second new element, radium. Even their relatively crude sample of radium was sixty times more radioactive than uranium. Eventually, it was found that pure elemental radium was two million times more radioactive than uranium.

This was the dawn of a new era. In 1903, Pierre and Marie Curie, together with Becquerel, were awarded the Nobel Prize for physics for their work on radioactivity. In 1904, Pierre was killed in an accident and the new chair in physics created at the Sorbonne, which was originally offered to Pierre, was given to Marie. She became the first woman professor and chairperson of a university department in France. In 1911, Marie was awarded a second Nobel Prize, this time in chemistry, for her discovery of the elements polonium and radium. Her eldest daughter, Irene, also became a Nobel laureate in physics. Both Marie and Irene eventually died of leukemia, probably as a result of radiation exposure.

Almost immediately after the discovery of radium, it was used to treat cancer. To begin with, only superficial cancers of the skin, lip, and other accessible sites were treated, with surprisingly good results. In 1903, Alexander Graham Bell wrote to a physician in New York, suggesting that "there is no reason why a tiny fragment of radium sealed up in a fine glass tube should not be inserted into the very heart of a cancer, acting directly on the diseased material." His idea was soon taken up and ushered in a new era of radiation therapy. Radioactive implants were soon used to treat cancer of the cervix with dramatic results. Even seriously advanced disease responded, sometimes with complete cure of the disease.

In the 1900s, the amount of radium available was very limited and a single gram of the element was valued at $100,000, a huge amount of money in those days. Fortunately, a mineral was discovered in Colorado that could be processed to supply more of the miraculous material. The Johns Hopkins Hospital, in Baltimore, became involved in procuring more of this mineral to ensure a supply for treating cancer of the cervix in its gynecology wards. Today, intra-cavity radiation is still used to treat cervical cancer, though other radioactive elements such as cesium and iridium have replaced radium. These newer materials are easier to seal and do not give off radioactive gases as does radium.

Radiation therapy has now become a very sophisticated science. The typical modern instrument used is the linear accelerator, in which electrons are accelerated to nearly the speed of light and when they hit a target, very high energy x-rays are emitted. These instruments were first created in 1953 in the United Kingdom. The first American linear accelerator is now on display at the Smithsonian Institution in Washington D.C.

CHEMOTHERAPY

With the advent of modern surgery and radiotherapy, only the last of today's trio of cancer treatment modalities was missing toward the middle of the twentieth century: chemotherapy. As in the case of x-rays and radium, serendipity played an important role, although the discovery of chemotherapy was also a cautionary tale of potential environmental disaster, involving biological and chemical weapons.

The idea of chemical drugs was not new. Paul Ehrlich coined the term *chemotherapy* to mean chemically derived targeted drugs that could be used against infections. Indeed, Ehrlich thought of tumors as being the result of "aberrant germs." It was therefore natural to use the term *chemotherapy* to mean drugs against infectious diseases as well as cancer. The development of chemotherapy against syphilis was accomplished in Ehrlich's laboratory in 1909 by screening a large number of organic arsenic compounds and isolating the efficacious compound, which he called Salvarsan. In 1908, he was awarded the Nobel Prize for his pioneering work in immunology, which was only one of his many contributions to medicine. Further success came in the 1930s and 1940s, in the form of sulfonamides and antibiotics as chemotherapy for pneumonia, meningitis, tuberculosis, and other common infections. However, the discovery of cancer chemotherapy had to await an unexpected event.

In November 1939, an explosion occurred on board a warship moored at the Italian port of Bari. The ship contained munitions, including chemical weapons, prepared for use in Second World War. Chief among the chemical weapons was mustard gas, a toxic gas also used during the First World War to devastating effect. A number of seamen on board were killed and many seriously injured. The incident was hushed up and many questions remain to this day as to what exactly happened, as most documents concerning the incident were classified as state secrets.

It was noted that among the survivors, many were suffering from a form of anemia characteristic of bone marrow failure. Pathologists performing autopsies on the dead seamen found that, not only was the bone marrow destroyed, but also the lymphatic organs were severely affected. From this macabre incident, several thoughtful young doctors made the deduction that substances related to mustard gas could be useful to treat cancers of the lymph and blood-forming organs. Despite the Official Secrets

Act, news of the disaster and the medical findings traveled fast. In 1941, a team of doctors at Yale University conducted a clinical trial of nitrogen mustard on patients suffering from lymphatic cancer. Their dramatic findings of regression of tumors were greeted with much excitement and many physicians followed their example of using mustard derivatives. However, it soon became clear that the remissions were temporary and the tumors inevitably returned. Nevertheless, the modern science of cancer chemotherapy was born.

The 1950s and 1960s were heady days of optimism in the scientific community. The defeat of Nazism and fascism brought new hope to the world. The crumbling of old edifices and the fall of em-pires transmitted a new confidence to the scientific world. Modern travel and modern communications eased the exchange of scientific ideas around the world. A number of chemotherapy drugs for cancer were discovered during this period. The mustard gas derivatives definitively established that toxic chemicals could be used to treat tumors, the trick being to find chemicals that, while effective, would not damage the patient too badly. This margin of safety was always set much narrower for these new drugs than it had been for other drugs, although by exploiting growth differences between cancer cells and healthy cells, a number of cytotoxic drugs were quickly developed and used to good effect.

Based on the principle that drugs for cancer should inhibit the growth of actively dividing cells, compounds that inhibit folic acid (a vitamin essential for cell growth) were developed in the 1940s and 1950s. With this advance in drug design came the first major clinical success—the eradication of a type of cancer that was previously fatal. The first cancer to be cured by chemotherapy was choriocarcinoma, a cancer resulting from malformed "moles" when pregnancies went wrong. Unlike cancers cured with surgery or radiation, which were localized tumors, these malignant moles had already spread or metastasized. This advance was hailed as a major breakthrough and the new drug, methotrexate, remains in use today. In 1948, Sydney Farber, a brilliant young Harvard pathologist and his colleagues reported temporary remissions in children with leukemia treated with methotrexate.

Armed with a few simple drugs such as methotrexate, mustard derivatives, a plant alkaloid called vincristine, and later some anti-tumor antibiotics, major forms of childhood cancer were beginning to be successfully treated. In the United States and other developed countries, cancer mortality among children declined by 50 percent, from eighty per million to forty per million of total population, during the past quarter of a century. This decline is mainly due to the dramatic improvements in the treatment for acute leukemia in childhood, one of the most impressive triumphs of chemotherapy.

In the 1960s, it became clear that two drugs were better than one, and three or more drugs were sometimes even more effective. With two or more drugs, an additive or even synergistic antitumor effect is present, and if the toxicities are different, the combination can be better tolerated. With this approach, children with leukemia sometimes survived two, three, or even four years, with repeated remissions and relapses. At St Jude's Hospital, in Memphis, Tennessee, in the 1960s, a team led by Donald Pinkel, Joseph Simone, and others carried out pioneering clinical trials involving hundreds of children. One hypothesis successfully tested was that, during remission, a few residual leukemia cells took sanctuary inside the central nervous system. Because of the blood-brain barrier, the drugs could not reach these cells. The team at St. Jude's therefore treated the nervous system of patients in remission with radiation and direct injection of drugs into the spinal fluid. The sanctuary hypothesis proved correct and a similar approach was soon adopted at other centers around the world. During the late 1960s and early 1970s, the cure rate for acute lymphoblastic leukemia (ALL) in children improved to 50 percent or higher. With further innovations in diagnosis and intensive treatment, the cure rate is now approximately 80 percent.

THE DISCOVERY OF DNA

The British physicists Sir William Bragg and his son, Lawrence, working mainly in Cambridge, laid the foundations that would eventually lead to the discovery of the structure of DNA. They worked on x-ray crystallography, a method of using x-ray diffraction to study the structure of crystals. In 1915, they became the

only father and son team to share a Nobel Prize. After the Second
World War, a number of young researchers converged on Cambridge.
Rosalind Franklin did her doctoral thesis there and went on to
work at King's College in London, where she made excellent x-ray
crystallographic studies of DNA. Many in the scientific community thought that she should have shared the Nobel Prize awarded
in 1962 for the discovery of DNA. Unfortunately, however, she
died of cancer in 1958 at the age of 38.

The gifted Austrian scientist Max Perutz studied chemistry in
Vienna and, in 1936, went to Cambridge to study for a Ph.D. on
crystallography. A year later, he found that hemoglobin, the red
pigment of blood cells, gave excellent x-ray crystallographic pictures. However, his work was interrupted by the Second World
War, during which he was interned as an alien. From 1947, he
directed a unit of the Medical Research Council, in Cambridge. At
first, the unit consisted only of Perutz and his assistant, John
Kendrew, and was located at the Cavendish laboratories headed
by Lawrence Bragg. Soon, this became the Molecular Biology
Laboratory and the focus of world talents, including Sydney Brenner, Francis Crick, James Watson, Cesar Milstein, and Frederick
Sanger, all of whom, as well as Perutz and Kendrew, were to
become Nobel laureates.

In 1951, Francis Crick and American biologist James Watson,
then only 23 years old, began their celebrated collaboration at the
Molecular Biology Laboratory. Their personalities were highly complementary and their great enthusiasm for scientific modeling soon
bore fruit, especially after they were given the x-ray crystallographic data of Rosalind Franklin, apparently without her author-
ization. These x-ray pictures were of very high quality, confirming
a structure for DNA consistent with the double helix model proposed by Crick and Watson in 1953. The double helix explained
how genetic messages could be coded in DNA and how DNA
could be replicated, with each strand of DNA forming a template
for the synthesis of a complementary strand. In 1961, another talented team of biologists, Jacques Monod, André Lwoff, and
François Jacob, showed how the coded instructions could be transmitted via another nucleic acid (messenger RNA) from the nucleus to the cytoplasm of the cell, where the instructions to make a

specific protein could be carried out. Thus, the most momentous discoveries in the history of science rapidly followed one another, completely transforming our understanding of the basis of biology and genetics.

Another major discovery at Cambridge was that of monoclonal antibodies by Cesar Milstein, an Argentine biologist, and his collaborator, Georges Kohler. These scientists made hybrid cells by fusing together mouse antibody-producing cells and cells from an immortal cell line developed from patients with cancer of the bone marrow. The technology enabled large quantities of a single antibody to be produced and is one of the first major applications of biotechnology to medicine.

MODERN LEUKEMIA TREATMENT

The treatment of leukemia (cancer of the blood), in particular, has been transformed by these scientific discoveries. A more thorough description of leukemia will help to explain how these seminal events are translated into the everyday medical treatment of a potentially deadly disease. Traditionally, leukemia is classified into four groups, according to whether it is acute or chronic and whether the disease involves lymphocytes of the immune system or blood cells other than lymphocytes. This traditional system remains a useful starting point to talk about leukemia today, although from a scientific standpoint it is superseded by classifications based on the genetic changes of the leukemia cells. From this classification system, we have acute lymphoblastic leukemia (ALL), acute myeloid leukemia (AML), chronic lymphocytic leukemia (CLL), and chronic myeloid leukemia (CML). The adjectives acute and chronic apply to the natural courses of untreated disease and originated more than half a century ago, reflecting the relative lack of capability to treat leukemia at the time. We now know that acute leukemia, although pursuing a rapid course, can in many cases be completely cured, and that some chronic (slowly progressive) leukemias, especially CML, require prompt treatment in order to arrest progression of the disease. Modern diagnostic methods, such as the study of chromosomes, have revealed that there are many more variants of leukemia, particularly subtypes of AML and ALL, which have their own distinct prognosis and mandate individualized strategies. Nonetheless, the appellations ALL, AML, CLL, and CML remain clinically useful and constitute a good framework for discussion of leukemia.

Most childhood leukemias are of the ALL type and the diagnosis is usually made by a bone marrow examination. This is done by withdrawing a small amount of the soft marrow, using a needle and syringe, from the pelvic bone. Children tolerate the procedure surprisingly well, and many children undergo bone marrow examinations forty times or more during the course of treatment and follow-up visits.

The abnormal cells in the bone marrow are analyzed to confirm the presence and type of leukemia. Tests using monoclonal antibodies and laser devices, plus chromosome analysis, enable the treatment team to ascertain vital information as to the subtype and whether the disease naturally has a good prognosis with standard treatment. For patients with more aggressive diseases, a more intensive strategy, such as the use of bone marrow transplantation, may be employed.

Treatment of leukemia generally falls into three phases. During the first phase, a combination of chemotherapy drugs is given to destroy the abnormal cells as rapidly as possible. When about 99 percent of the malignant cells have been destroyed, there is usually a return of healthy bone marrow function. Blood cells return to normal levels and an examination of the bone marrow using a microscope may not detect the small number of abnormal cells still present. This apparent return to normality is called a "remission"— this marks the end of the first phase. In the second phase, called "consolidation," the aim is to destroy the remaining malignant cells. As already described, some of these cells may hide in sanctuary sites, such as the central nervous system and the gonads. In children with ALL and some with AML, preventive treatment of potential disease in the brain and the spinal canal (and occasionally other sites) is usually given. However, the side effects of this treatment, such as possible impairment of intellectual growth, have to be carefully balanced against the potential benefits. This is where the analysis of good or poor prognosis subtypes and carefully performed clinical trials comparing long-term results of different treatments are particularly helpful.

The third phase consists of maintenance therapy, which may last for as long as two years for ALL, although less for AML. If there is a relapse of leukemia, very often a second remission can be induced. At this point, a decision may be made to perform a bone marrow or blood stem cell transplantation if a suitable donor is available. The overall cure rate for childhood ALL is now close to 80 percent, but is somewhat less for AML. For adults with ALL and AML, approximately 30 percent of patients may be cured with chemotherapy, with an additional 20 percent cured by transplantation.

For CML, major advances include transplantation and, most recently, a new drug called imatinib, which precisely targets the genetic abnormality of the malignant cells. The treatment of CLL is in a state of flux as new reports emerge of efficacy using a combination of three drugs, one of them a monoclonal antibody against a receptor called CD20 on the cell surface. The therapeutic use of another novel antibody alemtuzumab may also have tipped the optimal strategy toward attempting a complete cure of CLL. These promising reports have yet to be confirmed by further study. Meanwhile, the conventional recommendation remains to treat CLL only if it has gone beyond the early stage of disease.

Childhood leukemia, once a tragic and uniformly lethal disease, is now eminently treatable. Even so, most parents and the young patients themselves are stunned by the diagnosis of leukemia. In many centers, a dedicated team of specialist nurses, psychologists, and social workers help the family to cope with the devastating news, even when there is a good prospect of cure following intensive and often invasive treatments, as these often mean major disruptions to the lives of parents and siblings in addition to difficulties in adjusting school classes, sports, and other interests. Support groups, often including the families of other patients with leukemia, can be extremely valuable.

THE PROMISE OF BIOTECHNOLOGY

The most important driving force in our approach to the treatment of cancer in the new millennium is biotechnology. The power of biotechnology lies in its ability to replicate, on an industrial scale, many of the delicate scientific experiments performed on living cells. The products of biotechnology include drugs made by recombinant DNA technology, monoclonal antibodies, and cultured living cells as therapeutic agents made in clinical manufacturing facilities.

Genetic engineering, more formally known as recombinant DNA technology, allows scientists to isolate specific genes from one organism—for example, the segment of human DNA for insulin—and insert these genes into the DNA of another organism, such as a bacterium. This is done by first taking a ring of the bacterium DNA (a plasmid), which is cut at specific sites with an enzyme. A gene for the desired protein, such as insulin, is cut with the same enzyme and inserted into the plasmid, fitting the space exactly. The new DNA is said to be recombined or recombinant and is returned to the original bacterium. When the bacterium divides, the new genetic information enables it to make many copies of the gene, which directs it to make the desired protein.

Very large numbers of the modified bacteria can be grown in bioreactors under modern good manufacturing practice (GMP) standards, producing insulin, blood clotting factors, growth factors, and much more. Apart from bacteria and yeast, cultured mammalian cells can also be used to produce the desired proteins. It is also feasible to insert human genes into animals such as goats or rabbits. These "transgenic" animals can be programmed to produce the desired drugs, such as clotting proteins, in their milk. Commonly used anticancer drugs produced using recombinant DNA technologies include the T cell growth factor interleukin-2 and interferon.

A future possibility is the production of genetically modified cancer vaccines with specific directions to the immune system to recognize cancer cells. For example, "anti-idiotype" vaccines can be produced against cancers involving cells of the immune system, since individual clones of cells carry very specific markers or idiotypes. Such anti-idiotype vaccines have already shown promise in clinical trials for patients with malignant lymphoma.

When all the antibodies of a given batch are identical, they are said to be "monoclonal." Each batch of monoclonal antibodies is produced by a single clone of B cells, immune cells originating from the bone marrow with the specific function of secreting antibodies. If we have large numbers of identical copies of the specific antibody, these can home in on the specific cells. This is therefore a very powerful technology. To produce monoclonal antibodies, scientists use a hybridoma, meaning a hybrid cell. A hybridoma is a fusion of two cells. First, an animal, usually a mouse, is stimulated by the injection of an antigen and develops an antibody directed against it. It is then possible to isolate a secreting cell from the mouse immune system called a plasma cell, which is programmed to produce the antibody. This mouse plasma cell is then fused with a long-lived human plasma cell derived from a tumor of the bone marrow, a cancerous antibody-producing cell. The result is a hybrid cell that has the properties of secreting the desired antibody and of growing indefinitely. By continuous cell culture, very large numbers of the fused cells can be produced, each one producing the antibody specified by the immune cell.

Alternatively, completely human antibodies can be produced using a sophisticated methodology called phage display technology, a phage being a virus-infected cell engineered to required characteristics. The ready supply of these materials has revolutionized medicine, since all living cells have membrane receptors that can be readily recognized by these antibodies. The use of monoclonal antibodies in cancer treatment is a large and rapidly progressing field.

Biotechnology can also deliver large numbers of living cells with very specialized applications in the treatment of cancer. The cells may be obtained from the bone marrow or tissues such as lymph nodes, and sometimes from the tumors themselves. Cells can also be conveniently collected directly from blood using the technique of apheresis. Cells can also be grown in the laboratory, enhancing specific functions and increasing their numbers in a technology called ex-vivo expansion. These exciting developments offer great promise for the future, not only for the treatment of cancer but for other chronic diseases as well.

2

What Is Disease?

nderstanding the medical tradition from another culture presents many challenges. Not only is the pattern of diseases different due to geographical and economic factors, but also the very concepts of "disease" and "illness" can be radically different. Even within any one culture, these concepts can change greatly over a relatively short span of time. What do we mean when we say that someone has a disease or that she is ill? We may say of someone, "He's got cancer but he is not feeling ill." Or we may say "She is feeling sick" meaning that she has a hangover, but does not have a particular disease.

What do we mean when we talk about alternative, complementary, or integrative medicine in the context of a particular disease, such as cancer? Do we mean an alternative view of what constitute disease and illness, or do we mean only an alternative modality of treatment, in the way that radiotherapy and chemotherapy sometimes constitute alternatives for a given case of cancer? Are the treatment modalities truly complementary, such that some dietary supplements may ameliorate the side effects of chemotherapy? Or are the ways we think of "disease" complementary? For example, that cancer may be understood both as a mutation of the cancer cell's DNA and as a lack of healthy balance between life forces, the *yin* and the *yang*. By joining the two disparate viewpoints, can something new be gained? Perhaps we mean some or all of these things.

When it comes to "integrative" medicine, things are even more complicated, in part because the term *integrative medicine* arose out of political correctness. What this usually means in the West is that a tiny parcel of, say, Chinese medicine, is added as a token to a program constituted predominantly of conventional "mainstream" medicine. But in China, of course, this could be the other way around.

THE WESTERN CONCEPT OF "DISEASE"

The modern Western concept of "disease" is of relatively origins. European thinkers, particularly René Descartes (1596–1650), Sir Isaac Newton (1642–1727), and Charles Darwin (1809–1882), shaped our ideas of how the solar system, the planet Earth, and finally the cells and DNA of human beings work. The European Enlightenment gave us the framework of a universe as a mechanism, and then medicine itself changed. But because some of this understanding, particularly of genetics, is relatively recent, modern "scientific medicine" is a very new invention.

If we go back 100 years, or even to the time when the authors of this book were medical students in London and Paris, the idea of human diseases as purely mechanical problems, rather like a car with a broken gearbox to be treated with "spare part replacement," was still very novel. Indeed, the Western tradition from the time of Hippocrates (c. 420 BC) to William Harvey on the circulation of the blood (1628) followed a similar trajectory to the Chinese tradition over a similar period: from the herbal classic *Pen T'sao* (c. 200 BC) to the introduction of Western medicine in China about 200 years ago.

Throughout this period, the quest for knowledge was intense but was also beset by the lack of understanding of a unifying biological science. This was a noble search for truth as Aristotle described it:

> The investigation of the truth is in one way hard, in another easy. An indication of this is found in the fact that no one is able to attain the truth adequately, while on the other hand no one fails entirely, but everyone says something true about the nature of things, and while individually they contribute little or nothing to the truth, by the union of all a considerable amount is amassed.

In Europe, we only have to go back a little in time to find historical evidence of major epidemics being considered a form of divine punishment or of healing taken to be a miracle, a completely different view from the modern scientific approach. There is a famous painting by Goya called "The Procession of the Flagellants" (1816), which depicted holy men mortifying the flesh as a collective penitence. There is giant mural in the Great Hall of St Bartholomew's Hospital, one of the most famous teaching hospitals in England, by William Hogarth, depicting Christ curing a cripple. These themes continue today, although much diminished, in the way we experience suffering.

"DISEASE" IN CHINESE CULTURE

The fact that modern Western "scientific medicine" has not completely taken hold in China is probably not due to any inherent Chinese resistance to scientific methods, it may be simply a question of time, although the strength of Chinese culture has something to do with traditional Chinese medicine's ability to co-exist with Western medicine.

China is one of the most remarkable civilizations on this planet. There is less of an idea of mind-body separation in Chinese culture and especially in its medical culture. This influences the Chinese view of disease and health. In the modern West, a "healthy" person is like an expensive Swiss watch, all its mechanical parts in perfect order. The mind, however, is not fully understood in scientific terms. It is, in Arthur Koestler's (1905–1983) memorable phrase, the "ghost in the machine."

In China, particularly within that part of its culture that is heavily influenced by Buddhism, the human condition is fundamentally characterized by suffering and therefore does not have the imagined pristine quality that is idealized in the West. We find an echo of the Buddhist idea of suffering as a hallmark of the human condition in the work of existentialist writers in the West, such as Fyodor Dostoyevsky (1821–1881), Franz Kafka (1883–1924), and Albert Camus (1913–1960).

Through millennia, Chinese culture has been based on the three teachings: Confucianism, Taoism, and Buddhism. While Confucianism has been mainly involved in the development of the government bureaucracy, such as the appointment of court physicians and a system of apprenticeships, Buddhism and Taoism have had a more profound impact on the development of principles that underpin traditional Chinese medical thinking. A predominantly Buddhist tradition of medicine has in fact survived in the form of Tibetan medicine, which remains an important part of Chinese medicine. At its height, the kingdom of Tibet occupied almost one third of the geographical area of modern China. Much of this area is also very rich in herbs and continues today to be a major source of herbal medicines sold throughout China and around the world.

Influence of Buddhist Concepts

How does Buddhism view disease? Briefly, disease is viewed as an inevitable condition of human existence, because that existence is part of the realm of desire. In *The Teachings of Vimalakirti,* a popular sacred text of Mahajana Buddhism, the bodhisattva (holy man) Vimalakirti describes the body and its illnesses thus:

> Friends, he said to them, the body is transitory, fragile, unworthy of trust and weak. It is insubstantial, perishable, lasts for a short while, full of suffering, full of sickness and subject to change. And so my friends, the body, being the receptacle of so much sickness, knowledgeable people place no reliance on it.

According to the Buddhist idea, suffering—the Sanskrit word *duhkha* is sometimes rendered as "bitterness" or "the bitter sea"—has causes, and removal of the causes will result in the removal also of suffering. The suffering is therefore not inherent in human existence, only in human ignorance of the true reality. In Buddhism, the causes of *duhkha* are desire or greed, anger or hatred, and ignorance (in the sense of an incorrect appreciation of reality). In Tibetan medical tradition, the physicians, usually monks, are taught this view of suffering.

To illustrate: a beautiful young woman, perfectly made up, dressed in exquisite clothes, and wearing heaps of expensive jewelry, rushes out of a palatial home in tears, followed shortly by an obviously powerful and wealthy man—her husband. But her husband did not know which way she went, so he asked a monk standing nearby with his begging bowl: "Did you see a beautiful young woman, perfectly made up, dressed in exquisite clothes, with heaps of jewelry pass this way?" The monk answered: "I saw a pair of teeth went by." What a difference in the appreciation of reality!

The problem with the young couple can be summarized in one word—*duhkha,* suffering due to greed, anger, and ignorance. Greed for beautiful clothes and jewelry, even for beauty itself; anger because they probably had a quarrel, perhaps due to jealousy; and ignorance of the real facts of existence, that all will pass away quickly enough. Thus, this Eastern parable does not deny the mechanical facts of the case, the molecular biology of the beauty, or the design and workmanship of the clothes and jewelry. It simply denies that these mechanical "Swiss watch" attributes have anything to do with happiness. As with happiness, so with health.

Of course, a physician generally does not say to his patients: "You have an incorrect appreciation of reality" or "You are suffering from greed, anger, and delusion" or, even worse, "You have this illness because of karma." However, very often that is what, in Tibetan medicine, the physician is specifically taught—that the cause of illness is greed, hatred, ignorance, and the effect of karma.

Influence of Taoist Concepts

Taoism has given us the ideas of *yin* and *yang.* There is a very common misconception about *yin* and *yang,* a misconception that stresses differences. This is because the popular mind, especially the Western mind, is fundamentally dualistic and thrives on distinctions: fat or thin, short or tall, black or white. In our everyday life, there is an endless stream of distinctions, but as the Buddha has said, "All distinctions are falsely imagined." So with *yin* and *yang,* as the two arise from a unity which itself arises from an even more primal simplicity, the formless. Or to put it another way, from nothingness comes the one, from one comes two, and from two comes "ten thousand things," that is, everything. Taoism is very difficult to describe because the use of words itself creates dualism, so it is said that "the Tao that can be spoken is not the true Tao."

Of course, the practice of medicine is not a form of philosophical debate, although it is informed by philosophy. So, in discourse with the lay public, the Chinese physician describes the external and internal causes of disease, which lays the foundation of the physician-patient relationship. The external causes of disease are irregularities of daily living, such as diet, lack of exercise, and sexual excess. These are often described in the traditional symbolic language of wind, fire, cold, heat, dryness, and dampness. Some of these descriptions have a psychosomatic connotation: fire, for example, can denote irritability, anger, and a hot temper. The internal causes of disease are the loss of a state of balance, which extends to the mind as well as to the body. As in the West, traditional Chinese medicine recognizes, for example, that depression can cause an impairment of the immune response.

There are certain patterns of disharmony that are frequently observed and may result from excesses or deficiencies due to an unbalanced lifestyle. It is the diagnosis of this pattern of disharmony and its root cause that forms the basis of the Chinese physician's treatment. There are numerous patterns of disharmony, but most traditional physicians work from approximately seventy-five patterns, with innumerable variations upon these. The patterns themselves rest upon eight principles: *yin* and *yang,* internal and external, cold and heat, and deficiency and excess. According to a classical textbook, *yang* excess exhibits itself in fever, impatience, bad temper, headaches, and high blood pressure. *Yang* deficiency, on the other hand, may manifest in night sweats, exhaustion, constipation, backache, and impotence. *Yin* excess is rarely seen but may show itself in fluid retention, lethargy, and excess mucus. *Yin* deficiency results in nervous exhaustion and tension.

EAST AND WEST

Eastern thinkers and modern science both agree that the universe is unimaginably huge and that the world of living things (what the scientists call the "biosphere") is but a tiny part of it. Buddhism talks of innumerable universes and endless eons of time, which are consistent with modern astronomy. Of course, there remains the possibility that there are other biospheres out there. In any case, human beings are numerically only a minority among the living things on earth, though it is the one species with the ability to destroy the whole planet.

The central problem as seen by both Eastern thinkers and Western scientists is the "anthropocentric fallacy," the idea that the universe is made for us. It is not. If an alien being—say, a physician—traveling the vast expanse of space came across our galaxy and by chance got to know the ideas in the minds of selfish human beings, he would think "What rubbish!" In the West, because of the greater consumption of the planet's resources, the illusion is sometimes created that human beings are the center of the universe. What is more, individuals begin to think of themselves as the center of a mini-universe around them. In the East, this illusion is more difficult to sustain, hence more emphasis is placed on life as suffering, although as consumerism takes hold, a similar grandiose illusion is also engendered.

Chinese medicine, ever since it emerged from early shamanism and superstition, has been a secular culture, whereas in the West medicine had for many years been under the influence of theistic religion. Even when it apparently became secular in the modern era, Western medicine is still secular in a different way. The old religious West was concerned with the individual soul, the saving of which was the great drama of life. In the new secular West, the soul has been replaced by the individual "self" crying for desire gratification. This is why we have consumer-driven health-care in the West. Unfortunately, it is coming to the East now as well.

3

The Dark Valley

U ntil the mid-1960s, relatively few doctors used chemotherapy to treat the so-called solid tumors, such as cancers of the
breast, lung, and digestive organs. The use of chemotherapy was mainly restricted to a few academic centers and to a small
number of diseases, such as leukemia, known to be highly sensitive to the new drugs then being discovered. Vincent DeVita, a
renowned clinical researcher and for many years the head of the
National Cancer Institute, was reported as saying that, in 1966, the
waiting room for cancer chemotherapy at his institute consisted of
two chairs outside his office. This was to change dramatically during the next decades.

In the early 1970s, at President Richard Nixon's instigation, new
laws were passed by the U.S. Congress establishing comprehensive
cancer centers, which eventually numbered about fifty. These cancer
centers would offer cancer treatments of surgery, radiation therapy,
and chemotherapy, with some additional units specializing in gyne-
cological oncology and childhood cancers. During the past two
decades, these specialized centers have almost always included
bone marrow or blood cell transplant units. Similar centers were also
developed in Great Britain, continental Europe, and Japan during
this period. The new policy was a welcome change and meant large
increases in available resources of personnel, equipment, and fund-
ing. The pharmaceutical industry became involved as a major part-
ner in the effort to "win the war." President Nixon himself used the
term "war on cancer" and many groups adopted the war metaphor.

A CALL TO ARMS

Perhaps because of our tribal origins, war imagery has a very powerful appeal, evoking courage, heroism, and glory, as in this verse from William Blake's poem "Jerusalem":

> *Bring me my bowl of burning gold!*
> *Bring me my arrows of desire!*
> *Bring me my spear! O clouds, unfold!*
> *Bring me my chariots of fire!*

At some point, the word *kill* entered the vocabulary of cancer research, not in the sense of cancer patients being killed by the disease, or sometimes by the treatment, but as "cell kill." Cancer cells were the enemy and the proportion of cancer cells being killed by drugs became a surrogate measure of success on the battlefield, much as was done in the Vietnam War, which was occurring at about the same time—numbers Vietnamese insurgents killed in the field versus bodies of American soldiers being brought home.

This call to arms coincided with a wave of scientific developments in which the science of cell growth was studied using mathematical models, so it was natural to apply similar models to cell kill. Already in the 1950s, the new science of cellular proliferation kinetics developed concepts of the cell cycle, measured from the birth of a cell at cell division to its own division into daughter cells. Key events in the cell cycle at which a cell may, for example, decide to repeat the cycle or become a resting cell were being recognized. Howard Skipper, a cell biologist, had developed a proportional cell kill model based on mouse leukemia. This became a famous model but in reality it had no counterpart in human cancer—all the cells in Skipper's model are in continuous cell cycle, but in human disease the proportion of growing cells is sometimes relatively small. However, this and some other kinetic models of cell kill established useful general principles, for example, elucidating some causes of drug resistance. Another principle of drug development proposed at this time was the maximum tolerated dose (MTD), based on the concept of achieving maximum cell kill at the maximum dose tolerated by the host. Defining drug dose by toxicity became a standard practice in the treatment of cancer.

During this period of the rapid development of cancer treatment centers, especially in the United States, the "hawks" won the debate on the conduct of the war on cancer: more firepower, more cell kill, and higher MTD became the order of the day. From today's perspective, this emphasis on offensive weaponry was not a well-thought-out strategy, however. In human history, the side with the better defense has often emerged victorious. Indeed, this is true of many other facets of human activity; the games of football, chess, and bridge come to mind. In applying the war metaphor to cancer, the less glamorous work on the role of the immune system in this disease—the civil defense aspect of the war on cancer—received less attention. The result was a stalemate.

ARE WE LOSING THE WAR?

To gain a better perspective on the conduct of the war on cancer, we need to review some grim statistics. Three decades ago, in 1977, a report from the National Cancer Institute stated that twelve types of advanced cancer were curable to a certain extent using chemotherapy. That was indeed good news at that time. The curable cancers included several types of leukemia, lymphoma, testicular cancer, and some other rare cancers. Most of these advances were achieved before 1973. No new cancers have been added to the list for three decades.

In the United States, with the most advanced cancer treatment in the world, these highly treatable cancers accounted for less than 5 percent of all cancers. There were 44,500 new cases of these curable cancers in 1977, and 11,000 were cured with chemotherapy alone—slightly more than 1 percent of all cancers. In the eighteen-year period from 1973 to 1990, the cancer mortality rate in the U.S. actually increased by an annual rate of 0.6 percent.

According to the American Cancer Society, during the period from 1971 to 2002, among men, the annual deaths from lung cancer rose from 53,000 to 89,000, colon and rectal cancer increased from 22,000 to 28,000, and prostate cancer increased from 10,000 to 15,000. Among women during the same period, annual deaths from lung cancer rose from 11,000 to 66,000 (a six-fold increase), colon and rectal cancer increased from 24,000 to 29,000, and breast cancer increased from 31,000 to 40,000. In all, over 550,000 persons are expected to die of cancer in the U.S. each year.

The *Wall Street Journal* estimated the direct cost of cancer treatment in the U.S. alone at more than $60 billion in 1996; this has undoubtedly increased significantly since then. The indirect cost to society, in terms of lost production due to the illness itself or to depression among family members and other psychosocial upheavals related to the terrible disease, is harder to estimate.

In the words of Anna Akhmatova (1888–1966), the tragic Russian poet of the Soviet era, we have entered the dark valley:

> *Madness has already covered*
> *Half my soul with its wing*
> *And gives to drink of a fiery wine*
> *And beckons into the dark valley*

A pervasive sense of incomprehension and alienation set in. Cancer patients and their families began to ask: "Why is this happening?" "Is this indeed the best of all possible worlds?" "Can science do better?" Like Anna Akhmatova, who had seen her husband, son, and lover killed but who herself survived to criticize the Soviet regime, we should also re-evaluate the blinkered "more brute force is better" ideology of the war on cancer.

There is also the moral ambivalence in modern society when facing meaningless pain and suffering on a large scale. Western culture contains many examples of the alienation of useless suffering, which is discussed within a framework of moral and philosophical debate. An example of meaningless destruction of human lives was what followed an unexpected and devastating event that occurred in 1755. On All Saints' Day that year, as the inhabitants of Lisbon, the capital of Portugal, were at mass, there was an earthquake that destroyed half the city and killed at least 50,000 people. This was the subject of Voltaire's novel *Candide*. In this famous satire, the hero travelled to Lisbon with Dr. Pangloss at the time of the catastrophe. Among the falling masonry and corpses, the good doctor was found to be asking the question: "What can be the sufficient reason for this phenomenon?" Poor Candide can only answer: "The Day of Judgment has come." As they surveyed the devastation, Dr. Pangloss was moved to say: "All this is a manifestation of the rightness of things, since if there is a volcano at Lisbon it could not be anywhere else. For it is impossible for things not to be where they are, because everything is for the best." A little man in black, an officer of the Inquisition, who was sitting behind them, turned to Dr. Pangloss and politely said: "It appears, Sir, that you do not believe in original sin." This tale points to our ambivalence regarding the moral universe, whenever our search for the meaning of existence is met with indifference.

THE CASE OF LUNG CANCER

In cancer, despite all the efforts of the last three decades, there is despair among many sufferers and often among doctors and nurses who care for the patients. Voltaire's characters represented various perspectives, all of which were futile in the face of the destruction and suffering. For many doctors and nurses working in the field, a disease that typifies this sense of deepening gloom is lung cancer. Lung cancer used to be exceptionally rare: at the beginning of the twentieth century, doctors were sometimes taken specially to see a patient in the belief that they might not see another case in their professional lifetime. How ironic that now seems when lung cancer has become a scourge during the latter part of the last century and continues to be a monstrous killer.

The disease is occasionally discovered by chance as, for example, when an x-ray is taken for some other reason and a small shadow is found. Some of these early cancers are curable by surgery. Often, the disease manifests itself at a more advanced stage, with symptoms such as coughing up blood-stained mucus or shortness of breath. Sometimes, nonspecific symptoms such as poor appetite, weight loss, or pain may lead the sufferer to seek medical attention. Frequently, the manifestation might be due to the disease having spread to a distant organ, such as the brain, with the first sign being a seizure or even loss of consciousness.

There are several different types of lung cancer that are classified as belonging to one of two main groups: small cell lung cancer and all other lung cancers grouped together as non–small cell lung cancer. Small cell lung cancer is a very aggressive disease that tends to spread early, particularly to the brain and bone marrow. For the purpose of developing treatment strategies and guiding clinical decisions, a simple staging system is used, comprising only two stages, limited disease and extensive disease. Only rarely can small cell lung cancer be treated by surgery, so the mainstay of treatment is chemotherapy. Paradoxically, since the cancer cells are rapidly dividing, they are very sensitive to chemotherapy and the initial response rate is quite high, with some patients achieving a complete response.

This has led some researchers to apply the same principles that have been successfully used against leukemia—aggressive drug combinations, consolidation therapy, and treatment directed against malignant cells in sanctuary sites such as the brain, for example, by the use of whole-brain radiotherapy to prevent relapse. Even very high doses of chemotherapy followed by marrow or blood cell transplantation have been used to treat small cell lung cancer. The results have generally been disappointing, although a small proportion of patients with limited disease enjoyed long-term survival and have apparently been cured (the cure rate is less than 10 percent).

The majority of lung cancers belong to the non–small cell category, which is separated into stages according to the size of the primary tumor, whether it has spread to lymph nodes, whether the nodes of the opposite side to the primary tumor are also involved, and whether the cancer has spread to a distant site, such as the liver, bones, or the brain. The process of staging is performed using computerized tomography (CT) scans and often a direct examination of lymph nodes inside the chest (mediastinoscopy). Other diagnostic techniques, including blood tests, are performed. A positron-emission tomography (PET) scan is nowadays often used to detect very small amounts of cancer in distant sites.

After the staging is completed, it is usually found that approximately 20 percent of patients have stage I and stage II disease. These patients can be treated by surgery, but even then the chance of relapse is 30 to 40 percent. Most patients (70 to 80 percent) have stage III and stage IV disease. Stage III disease is further divided into stage IIIA and stage IIIB, the former is sometimes treatable with surgery, but the relapse rate is 50 to 60 percent. Most patients therefore have chemotherapy as a mainstay of treatment, although the improvement in survival with chemotherapy versus no chemotherapy is only about two to three months. Long-term survival or cure of patients with stage IV non–small cell lung cancer is an exceptional rarity. Eminent specialists with decades of experience in cancer chemotherapy interviewed for this book confirm that whereas, very occasionally, long-term survival is possible for disseminated cancers of the ovary, colon, or breast, they have not seen a single such patient with non–small cell lung cancer.

Lung cancer kills more than a million people every year worldwide, and accounts for approximately one-third of all cancer deaths. Yet, during the past three decades, there has been relatively little improvement in treatment outcome. Thus, lung cancer has accounted for 30 million deaths during this period. Compared to the major wars throughout history—we speak of the horrors of the battle for Verdun or the Nanjing massacre, each one with about 300,000 deaths—lung cancer is truly a major catastrophe and our current strategy needs to be examined further.

During three decades, tens of thousands of patients with lung cancer have been studied in chemotherapy clinical trials, mostly in the United States and Western Europe. In a recent article in the *Journal of Clinical Oncology,* a summary of results from the National Cancer Institute's database on thirty-three clinical trials performed from 1973 to 1994, comprising more than 8,000 patients, showed that comparing the period 1984–1994 with 1973–1983, the improvement in survival was only two-and-a-half weeks. Even then, some of the improvement may be more apparent than real since, in the more recent period, patients were more likely to have sophisticated scans and therefore may have been assigned a more accurate stage than in the past. That paper, not surprisingly, had the words "sobering results" as part of its title. In January 2002, the prestigious *New England Journal of Medicine* published an editorial entitled "Lung Cancer—Time to Move on From Chemotherapy."

Tobacco and Asbestos

In a paper on tobacco policy, Dr. Nigel Gray of the European Institute of Oncology, in Milan, succinctly stated: "The singular feature of the tobacco problem is that someone is selling it. No one is selling tuberculosis." Since the banning of asbestos, he is perhaps right about the "singular" feature.

Tobacco is a native plant of the Americas. There is archeological evidence that the Mayans were smoking the leaf as early as the first century BC. In the headquarters of the Imperial Tobacco Company, in Great Britain, there is a beautiful painting of a Mayan god enjoying a smoke. Christopher Columbus was fascinated to discover that the Arawak Indian tribe used dried tobacco leaves in their rituals and was offered some as a gift. Several of his men took up smoking and soon the habit was brought back to the Old World. However, smoking did not become popular until much later. In 1612, an imperial Chinese edict banned the growing or smoking of tobacco. Smoking was banned in Berlin in 1723. However, the invention of the cigarette-rolling machine in 1880 greatly boosted production, launching the modern tobacco industry, with its attendant hazards.

The eighteenth and nineteenth centuries saw the first reports of tobacco-linked cancers, such as cancers of the tongue or other parts of the mouth in pipe smokers, although, until the early part of the twentieth century, lung cancer was extraordinarily rare. Discovery of the link between cigarette smoking and lung cancer was also made difficult because of the usual lag period of twenty years or more between the onset of the smoking habit and the development of cancer.

In the 1920s and 1930s, some pathologists made the connection between cigarette smoking and lung cancer, but more definitive conclusions awaited the landmark studies of Richard Doll (who also linked asbestos and cancer and became one of the most prominent epidemiologists of the British Medical Research Council) and others. In Britain, both the Medical Research Council in 1957 and the Royal College of Physicians of London in 1962 published reports alerting the public to the serious health consequences of rising tobacco consumption and the evidence pointing to lung cancer.

The tobacco industry has been creative in facing up to the challenge of the scientific case against tobacco. It responded by advertising in television and other mass media. It planted smokers in films, sometimes paying actors to smoke on screen and developed marketing techniques using imagery suggestive of sexual prowess or associating the smoker to an adventurous personality. Until 2006, the tobacco industry sponsored Formula One motor racing. However, cigarette smoking began to decline in Western countries during the 1980s. So, the industry targeted youth and women in its media campaigns and developed a strategy focusing on exports to the markets of Asia, Africa, and Latin America.

The World Health Organization (WHO) estimated that tobacco would cause up to 10 million deaths a year by 2020. In the developed world, which has a longer history of cigarette smoking, lung cancer represented approximately 27 percent of tobacco-related deaths. In China, the percentage of lung cancer deaths as a total of tobacco-related deaths may be smaller, around 15 percent, but tobacco is also causally related to death from stomach and liver cancers. China's tobacco consumption more than quadrupled from 1965 to 1995, with serious public health problems likely to occur well into the middle of the twenty-first century.

After tobacco, asbestos is the second most widely manufactured carcinogen. It is a naturally occurring mineral that came into general use with the rapid pace of industrialization of the Western world in the nineteenth century. In the 1880s, large asbestos mines were developed, first in Quebec, Canada, and then in the United States, South Africa, and other countries. In South Africa, the mining of asbestos occurred in conditions closely resembling slave labor. During processing, the mineral rock was crushed to form a multitude of silky fine fibers. The best-known mineral was chrysotile, but other forms such as amosite and crocidolite were soon discovered. It was found that the fibers could be spun into textiles, thus launching a major industry.

As early as 1899, government inspectors in the United Kingdom singled out asbestos for its potential danger to workers in the industry. Indeed, even at the beginning of the twentieth century, researchers in the United States and Europe recognized the danger of asbestos because the very fine fibers could easily be inhaled, producing respiratory diseases. In 1931, the Trades Union Congress, in Britain, warned of a link between asbestos and lung cancer. Lung cancer was still a relatively rare disease at that time and the increasing number of asbestos workers with lung cancer was soon reported in the literature on both sides of the Atlantic.

In a foretaste of the response of powerful interests to the discovery of other carcinogens, the asbestos industry suppressed its own research findings. In March 1943, Dr. Leroy Gardner, a researcher for the industry, wrote to the National Cancer Institute: "In analyzing the results of a recently completed experiment on asbestosis, I was startled to discover that a small group of eleven white mice that had been inhaling asbestos dust for 15 to 24 months showed an excessive incidence (81.8 percent) of pulmonary cancer." However, a letter from the asbestos company Keasbey and Mattison stated: "We feel that reference to the question of cancer susceptibility should be omitted from Gardner's report since it is inconclusive." Gardner died in 1946 with his findings unpublished; the fruits of his labor were buried for three decades.

In the early 1950s, Richard Doll started to work on the relationship between asbestos and lung cancer. Together with John Knox, a researcher working for an asbestos company, Doll tried to publish the initial findings (the risk among asbestos workers was tenfold that of the general population) but was blocked by the company. Doll eventually published the data under his own name in 1955. Between 1961 and 1964, lung cancer accounted for nearly 55 percent of deaths related.

The association between asbestos and lung cancer might have remained insulated from public consciousness and governmental action had it not been for the discovery of a rare form of cancer called mesothelioma. This is a highly malignant tumor of the lining of the lungs for which there is no cure. Mesothelioma, once exceptionally rare, became the leading cause of asbestos-related deaths. In the late 1950s, a team of doctors and pathologists in South Africa uncovered a mesothelioma epidemic around the asbestos mines in Cape Province. One of the leading scientists of the group was Christopher Wagner. He and his colleagues not only firmly linked asbestos to mesothelioma but also pointed to the likely association of the malignant tumor developing with "neighborhood" or passive environmental exposure. The paper in the *British Journal of Industrial Medicine* was a bombshell. Soon, other reports emerged of clusters of mesothelioma cases developing in neighborhoods of asbestos factories or even among people living in asbestos-insulated buildings. In the public mind, the image of asbestos as a "killer dust" became firmly established. Even so, it took decades for asbestos to be banned in most developed countries as the industry fought a series of rearguard actions. In the United Kingdom, it was not completely banned until 1999. In 2001, the World Trade Organization concluded that there is no safe level of asbestos exposure, in that all types of asbestos are carcinogenic and that controlled risk in manufacture, use, and disposal is unachievable.

HOSPICE CARE FOR CANCER

With so many deaths from cancer, the revival of the hospice movement in the latter part of the twentieth century was timely. In the eastern part of the Holy Roman Empire, refuges for travelers were founded toward the middle of the fourth century. They were given the Latin name *hospitium*, derived from the word *hospes*, meaning "host," and the concepts of hospitality and caring continues to be part of the hospice movement today. During the Middle Ages in Europe, hospices proliferated to care for the needs of crusaders and pilgrims, especially the sick and wounded, and soon developed special skills for the care of the dying. However, in the fifteenth to eighteenth centuries, these special places of welcome and caring greatly diminished in number.

The movement was not revived until the nineteenth century, initially in Dublin, Ireland, and Lyon, France. Others soon followed and it was at one of those hospices, St. Luke's, in London, that a young woman, a volunteer nurse named Cecil Saunders, came to work in the late 1940s. She felt a natural calling to the care of terminally ill patients and was moved to make this her vocation. After taking a degree in medicine, she became medical officer for St. Joseph's Hospice, in London. In 1967, she founded the first modern hospice, St. Christopher's, in Sydenham, a suburb of London. This was the beginning of the modern movement combining the best of modern medicine with compassion for terminally ill patients, focusing on the needs of the patients rather than the "treatment" of diseases. For her pioneering work, Saunders was made a Dame of the British Empire.

In 1990, the World Health Organization defined palliative care as "the active total care of patients whose disease is not responsive to curative treatment" which "affirms life and regards dying as a normal process . . . neither hastens nor postpones death . . . and provides relief from pain and other distressing symptoms." Today, the hospice movement has evolved into a sophisticated approach with a dedicated team of professionals, including physicians, nurses, psychologists, social workers, physical therapists, and chaplains, usually available around the clock. Hospice care includes care in the patient's own home or at a day-care center, thus allowing terminally ill people to spend as much time as possible with their families. If a patient requires care in a hospital setting, this is made to be as much like home as possible. Volunteers are an important part of the team in the hospice movement. Thus, although a high proportion of cancer patients still die of their disease, they and their families, as well as the caregivers, have come to see dying as a normal process of change in which human dignity is preserved.

In the 1970s, the hospice movement crossed the Atlantic. Dr. Sylvia Lack opened the Connecticut Hospice in 1974 with a program to care for terminally ill people in their homes. During the following year, Balfour Mount opened the Palliative Care Service at the Royal Victoria Hospital, in Montréal, Canada. There was an obvious need for the type of service provided and, in less than two decades, more than 3,000 hospice programs opened in the U.S. and more than 700 opened in Britain. The movement has since spread across the globe.

A parallel development has been the pioneering studies by the psychiatrist Dr. Elisabeth Kübler-Ross on the subject of death and dying, beginning in the 1960s. Up to that time, this subject had been taboo. By studying the various stages of the dying processes, Dr Kübler-Ross brought into the open many of the unmet needs of terminally ill patients and their families at just the time that the general public was ready for a thorough discussion of the anxieties and fears associated with death and dying, which had been hidden for generations.

4

A Visit to a
Chinese Hospital

previous chapter looked at differences between concepts of disease and of the philosophy of medicine in China and the West. Here, we'll focus on the similarities, and it might come as a surprise to some readers that there is a great deal in common. Indeed, herbal medicine, as it is practiced in China today, is much closer to conventional Western medicine than either is to many forms of "alternative medicine" encountered in the West. This is because Chinese medicine, like Western medicine, is based heavily on empiricism rather than on the idea of the physician as a "faith healer" (at least not more so than is the case in the West).

Let us first look briefly at the history of medicine in China and visit a Chinese hospital in the city of Guangzhou, in southern China, where traditional and Western medical practices are fully integrated.

A BRIEF LOOK AT CHINESE MEDICINE

In Chinese folklore, the same legendary figure who brought agriculture to China, the emperor Shen Nung, also brought herbal medicine, around 2700 BC. Like primitive people everywhere, the early Chinese viewed illness in terms of animistic beliefs. In all of human experience, illness belongs with the larger categories of evil, calamity, and disorder. Like birth, death, and old age, illness is an event at once social and individual. In his search for the meaning of illness, early peoples first turned to explanatory models that attributed illness to beings—gods, demons, spirits, and ancestors. However, this shamanistic model was soon supplemented and largely replaced by empirical observations on the healing properties of herbs. By the time of the first historical medical text, the *Pen T'sao* (c. 200 BC), 240 vegetable herbs and 125 other remedies were recorded. In the ensuing centuries, more than 1,000 herbal medicines were added to the Chinese pharmacopoeia.

The subsequent development of Chinese medicine may be considered as having four interdependent aspects.

- First, there is a very large body of empirical observations, including clinical case histories, mainly of herbal treatment but distinctively Chinese modalities like acupuncture also became systematized and recorded. These are accessible through thousands of volumes of text.

- Second, there evolved over time a system of theories in which animistic beliefs and shamanism were replaced by a concept of health as a state of balance, involving both body and mind. It is fundamental to this philosophy that all life is in a state of flux, this being true of the world around us as well as of our bodies and our minds. Good health can only be restored through balance, according to this system of explanations. Seen in one context, this emphasizes preventive medicine. A seventh-century physician stated that "superior treatment consists of dealing with an illness before it appears; mediocre treatment consists of curing an illness on the point of revealing itself, inferior treatment consists of curing an illness once it has manifested." Superimposed on this theory of health through balance is an elaborate system of anatomical and physiological concepts such as channels for energy or *chi* (also spelled *qi*). Over the course of many centuries, the body of *clinical observations* (responses to herbal therapies and acupuncture) were correlated with the system of *explanations*. In modern China, however, many of the traditional explanations are being taught in parallel with, and occasionally set aside in favor of, scientific or Western explanations of disease. It is part of the Chinese genius that rival theories are well tolerated except during certain historical periods (the rise of communism being an obvious example of non-tolerance).

- Third, there emerged a system of cultural practices, such as dietary therapy and exercises to improve the *chi,* including Qigong and Tai chi, which are familiar to many in the West.

- Lastly, through the appointment of court physicians, a professional medical hierarchy gradually asserted itself.

Marco Polo arrived in China in AD 1275 and served for a time as an advisor to the court of Kublai Khan. In the succeeding centuries, Western missionaries brought with them medical knowledge from Europe, though this was, of course, not Western medicine in the modern scientific sense. The emperor K'ang-hsi, who reigned from 1662 to 1722, was supposed to have been cured of malaria by a Jesuit priest. In the nineteenth century, missionaries built and staffed many academic teaching hospitals in China, including the famous Peking Union Medical College in Beijing and Saint Mary's Hospital in Nanjing, which still exist today. These Western-style medical schools gained immense prestige as progressive-minded intellectuals in the late nineteenth and the early twentieth centuries turned to Europe and Japan for innovations in science, technology, and politics to bring China into the modern world. Sun Yat-sen (1866–1925), the founder of the Chinese republic, was himself a graduate of a Western medical school.

The People's Republic was founded in 1949. China was then still a vast, backward country, recovering from decades of war and civil war, with a rudimentary health-care system located mainly in the cities. In the countryside, it was hardly any different from a thousand years ago, with no doctors or nurses at all. People learned to pick their own herbs from the hillsides. During the 1950s and 1960s, a cadre of "bare foot doctors," minimally trained in public health and first aid, were sent to the vast hinterland to take care of the most basic medical needs of over one billion people. During the Cultural Revolution (1966–1976) the situation became even more chaotic and backward.

THE MODERN ERA IN CHINA

China began to modernize in earnest in 1978. Renowned schools of Western medicine in Beijing, Shanghai, Guangzhou, Hangzhou, and Nanjing were heavily funded by the central government and many new schools were founded. At the same time, academic institutes of traditional medicine were also expanded, their curriculum gradually incorporating modern Western subjects, such as anatomy and physiology, as well as traditional teachings about harmony and energy channels, while therapeutics continued to be based on herbal medicine.

Today, traditional and Western medicine are very well integrated in China. In 2004, traditional medicine accounted for 28 percent of health-care expenditures. But since the costs of consultations and prescriptions are less than corresponding items in Western medicine, the proportion of patient visits to the two types of practitioners are about equal, with traditional medicine playing a greater role in primary care.

China encourages the development and modernization of facilities where both traditional and Western medicine are practiced. These medical centers offer herbal medicine within a context of Western diagnostic technology. A typical such facility is the Guangdong Second Provincial Hospital of Traditional Chinese Medicine, in Guangzhou, a major city only a 90-minute train ride from Hong Kong. It is one of four affiliated hospitals of Guangzhou University of Traditional Chinese Medicine, one of the leading academic centers for traditional medicine in southern China.

Housed in a new squat, white building, it looks like any modern community hospital. The marble foyer opens onto a waiting area with comfortable sofas and signs directing the visitors to departments of laboratory, x-rays, computerized tomography (CT) scans, and magnetic resonance imaging. However, while the visual cues might be somewhat misleading, the olfactory cues are decisive—there is a distinctive aroma of herbal medicine coming from the pharmacy, which prepares over 1,000 individual herbal prescriptions a day. This is a hospital that plays by Western rules in regard to disease classification and clinical diagnosis, supplemented by traditional methods, such as taking the pulse. Therapeutics are, however, mostly traditional, with more than 600 different herbs available. Complex herbal combinations are prepared with the assistance of a computerized system. There is also a busy surgical department.

An Integrated Approach to Cancer

The hospital's outpatient clinics and inpatient departments see more than 2,000 new cases of cancer a year, mostly those that have failed to respond to Western treatments. Professor Lau Wai-sing, director of oncology, is a member of the standing committee of the China Anti-Cancer Society for Traditional Medicine and a renowned scholar. In his late fifties, Dr. Lau has the easygoing manner of a family doctor, is familiar with Western classification and staging of cancer, and can hold discussions on therapeutic outcomes based on complete and partial response rates and survival. He makes no exaggerated claims and does not think that traditional medicine can produce cures of advanced cancer, although symptoms can sometimes be palliated.

Professor Lau and his colleagues have a special interest in the use of the herb reishi (*Lingzhi*) and another fungus *Yunzhi* to help ameliorate the side effects of chemotherapy and to enhance anti-tumor immune responses. These herbs, together with *Cordyceps*, another fungus, are among the most commonly used to treat cancer. Chinese medicine, with its emphasis on healing through balance, is particularly interested in modulating the immune system to treat cancer, and these herbs are believed to act via innate immunity. Studies from the Chinese University of Hong Kong, which has a large cancer center based on Western medicine, showed that some *Yunzhi* extracts contain biologically active substances called peptidoglycans, which improve the lymphocyte (white blood cell) counts of immunocompromised subjects. These medicinal mushrooms are described more fully in subsequent chapters.

Another fungus, *Chaga,* is also commonly used in this hospital. *Chaga* has been used extensively in northern China to treat cancer. Mostly obtained from Siberia and not strictly speaking a traditional Chinese herb, it has been used for more than 400 years in Russia, Mongolia, and Korea. The herbs *Ginkgo biloba* and garlic are also used to help restore immunity. (These and many other herbal treatments for cancer are described in the major textbook *Management of Cancer with Chinese Medicine* by Li Peiwen, which has recently been translated into English.)

Many of the patients who attend the cancer clinics of the hospital have terminal cancer and have failed therapies elsewhere, so there is a very well staffed palliative care department. Acupuncture is used regularly in pain relief, an indication that is also increasingly accepted in the West. Many symptoms of advanced cancer can be relieved by herbal medicine, including anorexia, respiratory difficulties due to excessive mucus in secretions, diarrhea, constipation, and hiccups. The herbs used include Chinese hawthorn, licorice, Japanese honeysuckle, Korean mint, and many others.

In the same hospital, Western visitors will be astonished to find a fully functioning department of bone marrow and stem cell transplantation, representing the ultimate integration of Western medicine into a traditional Chinese hospital. The director of the program is Dr. Jiang Zhi-sheng, who previously directed a similar program in Nanjing and who appears to have seamlessly integrated his Western medicine activities into an environment where herbal medicine is the norm. Dr. Jiang, a member of the American Society of Hematology, explains that, in modern China, diseases that are eminently treatable by Western medicine, such as leukemia and lymphoma, are rarely treated with traditional medicine alone. Indeed, two of the most dramatic advances in Western oncology during the past decade—all transretinoic acid (ATRA) and arsenic trioxide for acute promyelocytic leukemia—were developed in China, though the main research was carried out in centers specializing in Western medicine.

As a social policy, integration of traditional and Western medicine is successful in China, where rapid economic progress has resulted in ever increasing demands for health care. It makes sense that the most effective Western medical advances should be introduced first.

5

A Success Story

ne of the greatest triumphs of modern medicine is organ
and tissue transplantation, which depends on understanding tolerance and rejection responses of the immune system. Transplantation of bone marrow stem cells has played an
important part in curing many forms of cancer of the blood and
lymphatic systems. Let us begin with a brief review of human
immune responses.

THE BODY'S DEFENSE SYSTEM

Living creatures share a potentially hostile world, teeming with a
bewildering array of infectious agents and foreign cells, so it goes
without saying that one of first requirements of life is some form
of defense. When speaking of the immune system, we generally
mean a complex system such as that found in human beings. Such
a system could recognize harmful germs or cancer cells. It is a system of learned responses that become stronger with repeated exposure to a harmful agent and are specific to that agent. For example,
once you have had chickenpox, your immune system will prevent
you from becoming re-infected because it recognizes the chickenpox virus and is able to destroy it. However, this response does not
protect against a different infectious agent such as measles, but
there may be cross-responses, such as a vaccination against cowpox that protects against smallpox. This type of response is called
adaptive immunity.

Unlike complex organisms, primitive organisms such as the horseshoe crab do not have a system with the ability to recognize specific harmful substances or cells. They do not possess learned responses but instead rely on "innate" immunity, which essentially mounts the same response whenever they face any danger. It took millions of years of evolution to develop the sophisticated human immune system, with its repertoire of billions of possible different combinations of recognition and responses. In addition to learned responses, such as that against chickenpox, human beings possess many of the defensive mechanisms of primitive creatures. In other words, humans have both innate immunity and acquired immunity.

An example of innate immunity is the acute phase response, which is mounted within minutes or seconds of contact with any harmful agent, whereas the acquired specific response typically takes weeks to develop. The acute phase response comprises a cascade of active proteins, one interesting example being C-reactive protein (CRP). For decades, scientists have known of the existence of CRP because its presence in blood dramatically increases upon contact with harmful organisms, sometimes as much as 1,000-fold during the first 24 hours after contact. However, the function of CRP was unknown until 1984, when scientists at Northwestern University, in Chicago, deconstructed the CRP molecule, which consists of five spheres linked together, and discovered that the single spheres or subunits are individually biologically very active. Research in animal models at the National Cancer Institute soon showed that the CRP subunits had anti-cancer activity, although this has not yet been confirmed in human clinical trials. The example of CRP shows that innate, as well as acquired, immunity may be important in preventing human cancer.

Immune System Cells

The immune system has the same level of complexity as the nervous system and is dispersed throughout the body. White blood cells called lymphocytes are the key components of the system and are deployed in special organs as well as circulating in the blood and in lymph, a milky substance that moves through its own channels (the lymphatic system). At intervals along these channels, aggregates of cells form lymph nodes. Other organs of the immune system include the tonsils and adenoids, the thymus gland (a small, many-lobed organ lying behind the breast bone), and the spleen, as well as patches of lymph aggregates in the walls of the small intestines.

The bone marrow, the soft tissue in the hollow center of many bones, is the site where many immune cells are produced. The two major types of lymphocytes are B cells and T cells. B cells produce antibodies whereas T cells, which include helper and suppressor cells, mediate a large range of cell-based responses. B cells are produced in the bone marrow and T cells originate in the thymus gland. The many subsets of B and T cells perform subtle immune functions, such as recognition of antigens and turning on and off specific responses.

An antigen is a substance, usually a protein or a peptide, which invokes an immune response. This may lead to the production of an antibody by the B cells, specific T cell responses such as production of cytotoxic T cells (which can directly kill viruses, bacteria, and cancer cells), or both sets of responses. However, the strength of the particular responses has to be regulated.

For a long time, scientists were puzzled by the opulence of the immune system with its ability to react to more than a billion antigens with responses individually tailored to each antigen. This amazing and apparently endless diversity is due to the ability of the immune system to "rearrange" genes. Generally, a gene is a segment of DNA with a fixed sequence for each of the body's functions; for example, specifying the structure of insulin. However, cells of the immune system are able to shuffle or rearrange many fragments of genes like a very large deck of cards. Typically, B and T cells are able to pick and choose among hundreds of DNA fragments for each cell's variable (V) region, diversity (D) region, joining (J) region, and constant (C) region of DNA. This apparently endless, though mathematically finite, ability allows the body to mount specific responses to a huge number of antigens.

THE DELICATE BALANCE
OF TOLERANCE AND REJECTION

A key function of the immune system is to distinguish between "self" and "non-self." In virtually every cell of the body, there are markers telling the body that it is its own cells or "self." For obvious reasons, the body's immune defenses do not normally attack cells and tissues that are recognized as self. This is called "self-tolerance." Interestingly, a fetus carrying antigens from the father (a distinct individual from the immune system's perspective) is also not rejected by the mother's immune defenses. Special mechanisms allow the immune system to tolerate the fetus, mediated by cells from both the fetus and the mother. Curiously, there is a certain similarity between the special privilege of the fetus and the mechanisms that some cancers have evolved to circumvent the natural defenses of the immune system. To overcome this undesirable immune tolerance of some tumors is an important challenge of cancer immunotherapy.

Therefore, tolerance and rejection are both essential functions of the immune system, modulated in a delicate balance in organ transplantation, which was introduced more than three decades ago and has become a widespread remedy for life-threatening diseases. For a transplant to succeed, the immune system of the recipient must be able to suppress its natural tendency to rid the body of the foreign organ. This problem can be tackled in two ways. First, the tissue of the donor and recipient should be as similar as possible. Tissue typing, or to use the technical term, *histocompatibility testing,* involves matching the markers of "self" on body tissues and has become a complex and sophisticated science involving immunology and genetics. The markers of "self" are called human leukocyte antigens (HLAs) and comprise sets of major antigens and minor antigens. Each member of a pair of antigens derives from each parent (maternal and paternal). "Self" and "non-self" are therefore not quite absolute, since tissue types among siblings are usually closer than among strangers, although even among siblings, some are a closer match than others. This is explained on the basis of genes determining the tissue antigens—we share more genes with some siblings than with others. The second approach to avoiding transplant rejection is to use powerful drugs to suppress the immune response. In practice, both approaches are often necessary. By fine-tuning these approaches, many transplant patients have been able to lead active lives, although the use of these powerful drugs to suppress the immune system is known to cause serious problems, including cancer.

THE SENTINEL CELL

For a long time, scientists thought that the immune system constantly patrolled for cancer cells and that cancer invariably represented a breakdown of immune defenses. This idea was first mooted in the nineteenth century by Paul Ehrlich and was restated in the 1950s by the Nobel laureate Macfarlane Burnett as the theory of immune surveillance. We now know, however, that this is too simplistic. To maintain health, the body must be able to tolerate a very large number of foreign antigens, so the immune system recognizes cells as foreign and stores the information in its memory. An active rejection response, in which the immune system marshals a large army of lymphocytes against invading bacteria or cancer cells, is in real life a relative rarity. The trigger for such a response is a sense of danger. This makes eminent sense, but how does the immune system recognize danger?

Paula Matzinger, one of the most charismatic figures of modern science, realized that despite the central role of recognizing "self" and "non-self" in immune responses, particularly in the field of transplantation, a more subtle response was required for everyday life. What the immune system needs to know when dealing with tens of thousands of foreign antigens each day is which of them are dangerous? One sign of danger is a type of unexpected or violent cell death, such as that caused by inflammation as a result of bacterial or viral infection. However, natural or programmed cell death (apoptosis) does not trigger the danger signal.

Distinguishing between reactions to the two types of cell death was a step forward, but the theory needed a special type of cell to fill the role of "sentinel." The dendritic cell (DC) filled the role perfectly. With many tentacle-like projections (dendrites), DCs have the appearance of mutant octopuses when viewed through a microscope. Since the mid-1990s, they have been the intense focus of immunologists. We now know that they are professional antigen-presenting cells and have very intimate contact with other cells of the immune system, especially T lymphocytes.

It is now possible to put the pieces together. A foreign antigen, perhaps a virus or a cancer cell, enters the body. The sentinel cell (usually a DC) encounters the antigen, digests it, and processes the information. It then has to make a judgment as to whether or not the antigen is dangerous. The sentinel cell undergoes a process of maturation and, according to the information it possesses (evidence of violent cell death or other signs of danger), will migrate to the lymph nodes and present the antigen to the T cells. A second signal, called the co-stimulation signal, is required to activate T cells and initiate an immune response in a very precise process. The co-stimulation signal is itself highly complex and delicately modulated and counter-modulated. This new field of knowledge holds much promise for the treatment of autoimmune diseases and cancer in the coming decades.

BONE MARROW TRANSPLANTATION

We now turn to the story of the transplantation of bone marrow stem cells. The practice of blood transfusion dates back several centuries, although it was initially conceived as an attempt to replenish an ebbing life force rather than with any true understanding of using blood cells as active treatment. Bone marrow transplantation is a more recent practice, its success a story of human ingenuity and tenacity. Marrow cells are dispersed throughout the soft cavities of the bones and function together as a blood-forming organ as well as an important part of the immune system. Accordingly, transplanting the cells of the bone marrow may accomplish the task of reconstituting the organ of blood formation (much as a new factory is built, in this case to produce blood cells). Transplantation may additionally be used to stimulate the immune reaction of donor cells to kill cancer cells in the host. To the pioneers of transplantation, these two uses of bone marrow were not conceptually separate. We now know, however, that of the two activities, the immune attack on cancer is the more important and is the first widely successful example of cellular immune therapy.

In 1939, a report appeared in the *Annals of Internal Medicine* describing a patient who had received a transfusion of bone marrow from his brother. This was the first attempt at bone marrow transplantation, opening up a new chapter in biological therapy (the use of living cells as active and specific treatment for diseases). Similar to other major advances described in this book, the discovery leading to successful bone marrow transplantation arose from chance observations relating to toxic exposure—in this case, radiation damage and its repair by the body. Casualties of the first atomic bomb explosions were extensively studied, including people who died almost immediately and those who developed blood diseases soon afterwards. Most of the casualties had severely damaged bone marrow. This led the experimental hematologist Leon Jacobson and his colleagues to report in 1949 that mice could be protected from lethal doses of ionizing radiation with a simple stratagem: the use of lead shielding for the spleen. Later, Jacobson showed that shielding the long bones conferred the same protection. This was soon followed by the discovery that transfusion of bone marrow had the same result.

During the next several years, researchers in the United Kingdom began an elegant series of experiments in mice, which showed that the protective effect was due to bone marrow cells that could repopulate the damaged marrow. These researchers further showed that cells from a different strain of mice conferred an additional immune effect against cancer. Thus, two key concepts were discovered during the 1950s. It became clear that there exist certain cells in the bone marrow and spleen (hematopoietic stem cells) from which all other blood cells could be derived. And it was formulated that a powerful immune effect ("graft-versus-tumor effect") could be developed as a treatment against cancer.

Clinical bone marrow transplantation in humans began with E. Donnall Thomas's pioneering studies in 1955. In the original method that remained in use for several decades, the technical aspects of collecting bone marrow were relatively simple. The procedure, called marrow harvest, was performed in the surgical operating theater. The donor had large numbers of punctures performed in the pelvic bone. Two doctors took turns to aspirate the

marrow with syringes. The aspirated material was manually fil-
tered through a stainless steel screen to remove particles of bone
and fat. It took up to two hours of drawing bone marrow before
the necessary quantity was obtained and placed in a blood transfusion bag ready for the recipient. With these simple techniques of
harvesting and infusing bone marrow, Thomas showed that the
procedure was inherently safe. While his initial attempts at treating patients were unsuccessful, he eventually overcame many of
the problems and his team became the leaders in this new mode
of therapy.

In 1959, George Mathé of Paris, another early pioneer, reported attempts to rescue victims of accidental radiation exposure with
donor bone marrow. Four of the five recipients survived, although
modern analysts suspect that at least some of the survivors had
limited radiation damage and the bone marrow recovered on its
own rather than through the transfused bone marrow cells. Mathé
went on to perform more transplants in patients with leukemia
and confirmed the power of the donor immune cells to kill
leukemia cells, although there was as yet insufficient understanding of how to manage the severe reaction against the host. All
except one of his patients died, most from the very powerful
immune reaction mounted by the transplanted bone marrow cells
against the host rather than the disease itself, as no trace of
leukemia could be found at autopsy. These early clinical studies of
patients with incurable advanced disease showed that powerful
immune reactions can kill leukemia cells (the graft-versus-cancer
effect) but they can also kill many of the host's healthy cells, including cells of the liver, lung, skin, and other tissues (the graft-
versus-host effect).

With the exception of transplants between identical twins
(one of which was performed by Dr. Lu Dao-Pei in Beijing, in
1964, the first such transplant in Asia), all clinical bone marrow
transplants during the 1950s and early 1960s failed because of
severe graft-versus-host effects. This did not affect Lu's patient
because identical twins naturally share their genetic make-up
and so there is no rejection in either direction. Both the patient
and her donor are still alive in 2005, more than 40 years after
the transplant.

Tissue Typing

The serious setback in the 1960s led the prominent scientist Dirk van Bekkum to say in 1966 that "many investigators had abandoned the idea that bone marrow transplantation can ever become a valuable asset in clinical medicine." For E. Donnall Thomas, it was back to the drawing board. He and other researchers realized what the major cause of failure might be: the difference between mouse and human models was that the mice were inbred and therefore genetically identical or closely similar, whereas humans were genetically diverse and rejection (in both directions) was a much bigger problem. It was therefore decided to study a large, random-breeding animal model and the obvious choice was the dog. A canine tissue typing system was developed in 1968. Immunosuppressive drugs were also developed, helping to moderate the graft-versus-host reaction. Using these drugs and total body irradiation to kill the host bone marrow, together with the newly acquired knowledge of tissue typing in dogs, Thomas and his team soon showed that canine bone marrow transplants could be successful among tissue-matched littermates. Thomas lived on a farm on the outskirts of Seattle at that time and, with the success of canine transplantation, he soon had more than forty dogs living on his farm.

After working out the tissue typing system in dogs involving dog leukocyte antigen (DLA), Thomas and others studied the human leukocyte antigen (HLA) system, which has since become universally adopted, with many known transplantation antigens. This system defines immune barriers for transplantation with different degrees of closeness or separation. Scientists have described these immune barriers, or transplantation antigens, which are coded by sets of genes. The most important of these antigens are called HLA-A, HLA-B, HLA-C, HLA-DR, HLA-DQ, and HLA-DP.

We inherit half of our HLA genes from our father and half from our mother. This means that, with the exception of identical twins, the chance of any given sibling having a complete HLA match is 25 percent. Bone marrow from an identical twin is obviously the ideal cell source, but this is available to very few patients in need of a transplant. Many transplants use cells from a sibling, matched for compatibility. A sibling with an incomplete match, such as one antigen mismatch, can be used as a donor, but if a sibling donor is not available, a search is often made for an unrelated donor. Nowadays, sophisticated molecular genetic techniques are available to ensure the best match with unrelated donors. Even so, the risks of transplantation using cells from an unrelated donor are significantly greater.

In 1975, Dr. Thomas was able to show that, even among patients with very advanced leukemia, transplants could cure some of them. Of the first 100 patients, 13 were cured. It was a great achievement, since nearly all of them were transplanted as a last resort, having failed all other available treatments. Many other clinical successes followed and, in 1990, Thomas received the Nobel Prize for medicine.

Finding Progenitor Cells

A transplant team has to accommodate patients with aggressive disease who may have to "jump the queue" to have any chance of cure, as well as patients scheduled for elective transplant in a timely manner. Often a donor has to be found among volunteers, possibly from overseas. Collection of bone marrow or peripheral blood progenitor cells is sometimes done thousands of miles away from the transplant center and conveyed there by courier.

Progenitor cells are those cells of the bone marrow that can indefinitely generate progeny of the different types of blood cells. We now know that these cells can also be collected from the peripheral blood if the donor is first primed with injections of blood cell growth factors, such as granulocyte colony-stimulating factor (G-CSF). After about four days of priming, relatively large numbers of progenitor cells can be found in the peripheral blood circulation. They can then be collected using a cell separator so that collecting marrow from the pelvic bone is no longer necessary, although it is still done for specific indications. From the standpoint of donor comfort and safety, collecting cells from blood is clearly preferable.

The process of stimulating the release of progenitor cells from bone marrow using injections of growth factors developed from genetic engineering is a major achievement of biotechnology. When we speak of someone having a bone marrow or blood cell transplant, we often mean a transplant using such cells collected from blood following stimulation with G-CSF. Apart from the peripheral blood, cells suitable for transplantation are also obtained from the placenta and umbilical cord. The use of cord blood stem cells in transplantation has now become a standard treatment for many genetic and blood diseases.

Fortunately, there is good international collaboration, with a worldwide registry of more than 200,000 voluntary donors of bone marrow or peripheral blood stem cells. There is also an international inventory of more than 300,000 units of umbilical cord blood. Worldwide standards have been established for tissue typing of donors and recipients as well as quality controls for collection and transplant centers. Even so, finding a match and arranging the logistics of cell harvest often takes several months, a critical time frame for someone with advanced cancer. In 2005, more than 200 teams performed approximately 50,000 transplants, not counting transplants using the patient's own (autologous) cells. There are transplant teams in North America, Western Europe, most of the countries of the former Soviet Union and Yugoslavia, and in many major cities in China, Japan, Taiwan, Korea, Israel, and other countries.

The Transplant Operation

Once a donor is found, the team will hold a conference with the participation of transplant physicians, scientists, psychologists, specially trained nurses, the patient and his family and, sometimes in the case of a sibling donor, the donor. During the conference, the process of transplantation is described in detail and the logistics discussed. The timing of the transplant is extremely important and depends on the nature of the specific underlying disease. For patients with high risk for relapse, the transplant is often carried out during the first complete remission, whereas for patients with a low risk for relapse, it is generally better to wait since a transplant may not always be necessary.

In most centers, the recipient is admitted to hospital 10–14 days before the procedure. A Hickman catheter is used for infusion of drugs and blood products and can remain in situ for several months. The patient receives high doses of chemotherapy given through the catheter and, in many cases, also undergoes total body irradiation. These treatments collectively are called "conditioning," and they prepare the bone marrow to receive the transplant.

On the day of the transplant, cells are collected from the donor using a cell separator or directly from the bone marrow. In the latter instance, the donor receives a general anesthetic. Donation involves minimal risk and a small degree of discomfort and recovery is generally rapid. The cells are then prepared in a blood transfusion bag and hung by the bedside.

During the next two weeks, the recipient receives intensive nursing care as there is lowered resistance against infections. Drugs are given to combat rejection and graft-versus-host disease and also to prevent viral, bacterial, and fungal infection. Growth factors are sometimes given to expedite the development of white blood cells from the bone marrow. For a conventional transplant, the recipient has to remain in the hospital for approximately one month, but the period is much shorter for a transplant involving reduced conditioning (these newly introduced procedures are commonly referred to as "mini transplants"). After discharge from the hospital, the recipient must be closely monitored for the first six to twelve months. However, most people who have received transplants eventually return to a near normal lifestyle.

Sometimes the patient's own cells can be used for what are known as auto-transplants. The cells are collected, sorted, and frozen in storage while the patient undergoes intensive therapy. This treatment modality is not strictly speaking transplantation but rather a re-infusion of cells. Because the process utilizes the patients' own cells, not only is there no need to look for a donor but it also confers a high degree of safety, since there is no possibility of rejection. Such transplants have been developed so that there is a minimal requirement for hospital stay. Many teams have performed more than 100 consecutive autologous transplants with no mortality. This strategy, which allows an intensive schedule of chemotherapy to be given, has become routine for some types of lymphoma and myeloma. However it lacks the advantage of the immune reaction of the donor cells against the tumor (graft-versus-tumor effect).

6

Nature's Healing Gift

Human beings have been using mushrooms as medicines for 5,000 years or more. As we shall see, many mushrooms have properties that can improve health and well-being. What we call a "mushroom" is the fruit-body of a fungus, the reproductive part that grows above ground and releases spores, the seed-like elements from which new fungus are made. Much as fruit is the reproductive organ of a fruit tree, a mushroom is the reproductive organ of a fungus.

Typically, spores sprout from the gills, the thin brown tissue found on the underside of the mushroom cap. Borne by the wind, some kinds of spores are capable of traveling great distances from the fruit-body to start their own fungus colonies. Mushrooms produce prodigious numbers of spores. A giant puffball, for example, may produce 20 trillion; it has been calculated that if every spore from the giant puffball sprouted and grew to maturity, it would form a mass three times the size of the sun! The spores are produced in such large numbers to guarantee the spread of the fungus in the environment. As mycologist Elio Schaechter has written, "Lavishness is necessary; rare is the spore that germinates into successful fungal growth. Such wastefulness, however, is not unlike the production of millions of unsuccessful sperm by the human male."

Not all fungi, however, produce mushrooms. Some are able to create spores and reproduce without bearing a fruit-body. Fungi that reproduce without a sexual stage are called imperfect fungi (*fungi imperfecti*).

THE GREAT RECYCLERS

In nature, fungi are the great recyclers. To feed itself, but also to assist plants in getting the nutrients they need, a fungus breaks down organic matter into essential elements. According to recent estimates by David Hawksworth, there are over 1,500,000 species of fungi on earth. Mushrooms constitute at least 14,000, and perhaps as many as 20,000, known species, but this may be less than 10 percent of the total. Assuming that the proportion of useful mushrooms among the undiscovered mushrooms will be only 5 percent, there may be thousands of as yet undiscovered species that will be of possible benefit to humankind. Even among the known species, the proportion of well-investigated mushrooms is very low. About 700 species are eaten as food, and 50 or so species are poisonous.

Fungi make up about a quarter of the biomass of the earth. They need organic matter to feed on, develop, and grow. Strange as it may seem, seeing that they are usually associated with rot and decay, fungi are something of a cleanser in that they transform organic matter into nutrients that plants and animals can feed on. Without fungi, matter would not break down and decompose, and the world would be crowded with dead animals and plants.

LIFE CYCLE OF THE MUSHROOM

Every fungus begins as a tiny seed-like spore. Spores are carried by wind and water. When a spore lands in a hospitable place—a moist place that is not too hot or cold and is near a food source—it may germinate and start a new fungus colony. At that point, the spore grows hyphae, the fine, threadlike strands from which the mycelium is made. The mycelium is the feeding body of the mushroom. Composed of a latticework of interconnected hyphae threads, it is for the most part subterranean, living in soil or decayed wood, much like the root system of a plant. It can feed on almost any organic substrate: soil, wood rot, or food left for too long in the pantry.

How fast and how large the mycelium grows depends on environmental factors such as soil temperature and the accessibility of food. Researchers have reported finding a mycelium beneath the soil of Michigan that is 1,500 years old and 35 acres wide and weighs 100 tons. This mycelium is from the fungus *Armillaria bulbosa*, a root pathogen of aspen. Using molecular methods, the researchers mapped the extent of the fungus genome to show that the mycelium germinated from a single spore.

The mycelium insinuates itself into the substrate on which it feeds and secretes enzymes. These enzymes break down organic material in such a way that the fungus can absorb food from the substrate. Research has shown that these complex enzymes act as a growth stimulus to nearby plants. They degrade organic material so that important nutrients are returned to the soil where plants can feed on them. In this way, fungi provide the raw material for trees and other plants.

Fungi are essential for a healthy forest. If there are no fungi in the soil, plants cannot grow because they cannot break down and absorb nutrients without the help of fungi. One group of mushrooms called the mycorrhizae attach themselves to the roots of trees. They act like a secondary root system, reaching deep into the soil to get nutrients that the tree could not otherwise get, and passing these nutrients upwards to the tree. In return, trees provide the mycorrhizal fungus with a set of nutrients that they need to grow. The fungus and tree work together in a symbiotic partnership, with some plant growth hormones produced by fungi. Many plants cannot survive without fungi.

In effect, fungi are molecular disassemblers: they take the complex compounds created by plants, such as cellulose, carbohydrates, and protein and disassemble them so that they can be easily digested. By contrast, plants are molecular assemblers, taking very simple compounds made of nitrogen, carbon, and sometimes water and combining them into complex forms such as protein, carbohydrates, and cellulose.

MUSHROOMS AS MEDICINE

Some scientists believe that the ability of mushrooms to break down organic matter in nature is linked to their medicinal properties for humans. Fungi live in a hostile environment, in the midst of decay, at the harshest layer of the ecosystem. They encounter disease-causing pathogens far more frequently than other life forms. To survive, they must have proactive, healthy immune functions. Some scientists believe that the anti-pathogenic properties developed by mushrooms as a survival mechanism are precisely what make them valuable to the human immune system.

In the distant human past, all plants and animals were seen as repositories of secret power that could be used for good or ill. In a sense, the whole world was a pharmacopoeia. Our ancestors' relationship to the food they ate was very different from ours. In our day, most people have lost the primal connection to the food we put in our bodies, and with it we have lost our connection to the earth. Mushrooms are potent medicines and contain many nutrients. When you take a medicinal mushroom you get back in touch with the essential forces of the earth. Humankind has benefited from the healing properties of medicinal mushrooms for centuries and we look forward to new discoveries by science to harness that medicinal power for the good of all.

Many claims are made for medicinal mushrooms. For this book, we have carefully examined sources of information to make sure they were reliable. Except for historical purposes, we have endeavored to cite only studies and experiments that were undertaken in the past decade in order to present the most current information about the healing properties of mushrooms. We will focus on scientific studies of the immune-modulating and curative properties of medicinal mushrooms. Most of these studies were done in China, Korea, and Japan. We believe these studies to be valid and the medicinal mushrooms used in them are increasingly being accepted in both the East and West. But no medicinal mushroom is a cure-all and no mushroom can make the body unassailable to disease. What they can do is stimulate the immune response, giving a powerful boost to the functions of the body that are already in place for preventing and fighting disease. This is particularly true for patients who have cancer.

AGARICUS BLAZEI

We begin with the story of *Agaricus blazei,* a relative newcomer to the exciting armamentarium of medicinal mushrooms. Many scientists believe that the beta-glucans in *Agaricus blazei* are more potent than those of other mushrooms. Beta-glucans are polysaccharides, or sugar molecules, thought to stimulate and balance the immune system. The main beta-glucan is the 1-6 form, shaped in a spiral somewhat similar to the famous helix of DNA. Forty years ago, only a few thousand villagers in Brazil knew of the medicinal properties of this mushroom, but since the world discovered the mushroom, its reputation has spread far and wide. *Agaricus blazei* has shown real promise as an immune modulator and a defense against cancer.

Instead of the exotic East, the origins of *Agaricus blazei* can be traced to a small mountain town in Brazil called Piedade, located 120 miles (200 kilometers) southeast of Sao Paulo. For centuries, the inhabitants of the town and its environs have savored a mushroom that they call *Cogumelo de Deus* ("mushroom of God"), *Cogumelo Princesa* ("Princess mushroom"), *Cogumelo do sol* ("the sun mushroom"), or *Cogumelo da Vida* ("mushroom of Life"). In the summer of 1965, a Brazilian farmer of Japanese descent named Takahisa Furumoto was roaming the mountains outside Piedade when he found an unfamiliar but tasty mushroom. The mushroom appeared to be of the *Agaricus* family. Furumoto sent spores of the mushroom to Inosuke Iwade of the Iwade Research Institute of Mycology, in Japan. To learn more about the mushroom, Iwade, a scholar in the field of mushroom cultivation, attempted to grow the mushroom in his laboratory, an attempt that would take nearly a decade.

Meanwhile, back in Piedade, a group of scientists led by Dr. W.J. Cinden of Pennsylvania State University had begun their own investigation into the unknown *Agaricus* mushroom. Dr. Cinden and his colleagues had come to Piedade to find out why the inhabitants of the town had low rates of geriatric diseases and a reputation for longevity. He concluded that the people of Piedade enjoyed long life because they were eating an unusual mushroom of the *Agaricus* family as part of their diet. He published his findings in *Science* magazine and presented his conclusions at several conferences. Word about the unusual mushroom from Brazil began to spread.

After Inosuke Iwade at last managed to cultivate samples of the *Agaricus* mushroom in his laboratory, he noticed that this mushroom was longer and thicker than others in the *Agaricus* family. The gills took longer than usual to turn black, the mushroom emitted a strong aromatic odor, and the root was sweet and delicious. Did he have a new species on his hands? Iwade submitted a sample of his mushroom to a Belgian taxonomist named Paul Heinemann, who deemed the mushroom a new species. He called it *Agaricus blazei* Murrill, after the American mycologist William Murrill.

Some cynics say that the story of the longevity of the inhabitants of Piedade has been invented and that in reality the people in that area had never eaten the *Agaricus* mushroom, which today is not even common in that area. William Murrill, so the story goes, had found the mushroom in the 1940s on the lawn of his friend R.W. Blaze, who lived in Gainesville, Florida. Murrill had discovered over 600 species of fungi during his productive life. However the case may be, it was in the 1960s that Japanese living in Brazil rediscovered it and Japanese companies have produced a variety of medicinal drugs based on this fungus.

Agaricus blazei favors the humid, hothouse environment of its native Brazil. It grows only in the hot summer months and it may die if the temperature drops too low. In the Piedade region, temperatures range from 35°C (95°F) during the day to 22.2°C (72°F) at night and the land receives a good dousing by tropical rain in the afternoon or early evening. According to a story, one reason that *Agaricus blazei* thrives in the region has to do with the number of wild horses found there. Horse manure, the story goes, contributes to the fertility and unique composition of the soil!

Clinical interest in *Agaricus blazei* began in earnest when a study showing anti-tumor activity of the mushroom was presented at a convention of the Japanese Cancer Association in 1980. In the study, *Agaricus blazei* was shown to have higher levels of beta-glucan than maitake, shiitake, or reishi mushrooms. Scientists believe that *Agaricus blazei* contains the highest level of beta-glucans of any mushroom. They are (1-6)-(1-3)-beta-D-glucans, polysaccharide-protein complex, RNA-protein complexes, and glucomannan. In 1995, Dr. Takashi Mizuno, who has studied *Agaricus blazei* for many years, isolated an active anti-tumor compound from the mushroom.

Scientists at Kobe Pharmaceutical University in Japan tested the effects of *Agaricus blazei* on cancer. They injected a water-soluble fraction of the mushroom into mice bearing tumors and a control group was injected with saline only. They found an increase in T cells in the mice treated with the extract. At the Mie University School of Medicine, in Japan, scientists found that *Agaricus blazei* also increased an important component, called C3, of the complement system, part of the innate immune system. Many other studies of this mushroom on cancer are now in progress.

MAITAKE

Maitake means "dancing mushroom" in Japanese (*mai* means "dance"; *take* means "mushroom"). How the mushroom got its name depends on which story you choose to believe. In one account, the mushroom got its name because people danced with joy upon finding maitake mushrooms in the forest. They may well have danced with joy during Japan's feudal era, when local lords paid tribute to the shogun by presenting him with maitake mushrooms, among other gifts. To obtain the maitake mushrooms, the local lords are supposed to have offered anyone who found one the mushroom's weight in silver, a cause for dancing indeed. Another story says that the dancing mushroom got its name because the overlapping fruit-bodies give the appearance of a cloud of dancing butterflies.

In the English-speaking world, maitake is known as "Hen of the Woods." The mushroom, growing as it does in clusters, is said to resemble the fluffed tail feathers of a brooding hen. Less frequently, the mushroom is called the more prosaic "Sheep's Head." It is sometimes called the "king of mushrooms" on account of its size. The mushroom's Latin name is *Grifola frondosa*. *Grifola* is the name of a fungus found in Italy. Some scholars believe that the fungus got its name from the griffin (or griffon), the mythological beast with the head and wings of an eagle and the hind legs and tail of a lion. *Frondosa* means "leaf-like" as the overlapping caps of maitake mushrooms growing in the wild give the appearance of leaves.

The chief characteristic of the maitake mushroom is that it grows in clusters. The caps, which are typically four to five inches across, overlap one another to form a sort of clump. The stems, meanwhile, fuse together. Maitake grows at the base of oak trees, beeches, and other dead or dying hardwoods. According to folklore, the mushroom prefers to grow where lightning has scarred the wood of a tree. A typical maitake cluster is the size of a volleyball, but some clusters can be twenty inches (50 cm) in diameter and weigh as much as eighty pounds (36 kg). The mushroom prefers temperate northern forests. It is indigenous to northeast Japan, Europe, Asia and the eastern side of the North American continent. Connoisseurs favor maitake mushrooms from Japan for their flavor.

Commercial techniques for the cultivation of maitake mushrooms were not perfected until the late 1970s. Before then, the only way to harvest maitake was to pick it in the wild. Foragers in Japan were said to be very covetous of the secret places where maitake grew. To mark their forest turf and keep others away, foragers cut hatch marks into trees. Known locations of maitake were called "treasure islands." Many a forager kept the secret his entire life and revealed it only in his will so that his eldest son could find his way to the treasure.

Since maitake cultivation is a recent development, only in the past two decades have producers been able to switch from a reliance on foraged maitake to offering cultivated maitake. Japanese commercial cultivation, mainly for food, started in 1981 with 325 tons. Commercial maitake production worldwide may now be in excess of 50,000 tons per year.

Maitake is a delicious culinary mushroom, but the Japanese also value it for its medicinal properties. Traditionally, maitake was used in Japan as a tonic to boost the immune system and increase vitality, and the mushroom was supposed to prevent cancer and high blood pressure. For that reason, researchers turned their attention to maitake's effects on those diseases when they first began experimenting with it three decades ago. In recent years, the maitake mushroom has become a popular subject for study. In Medline, the online database of the National Library of Medicine, there are more studies pertaining to maitake than to any other mushroom covered in this book.

In 1984, Japanese mycologist Hiroaki Nanba, of the Kobe Pharmaceutical University, identified a substance found in both the mycelia and the fruit body of maitake that had the ability to stimulate macrophages, an immune cell that destroys antigens. This so-called D-fraction is a standardized form of beta-glucan polysaccharide compounds (mainly beta-D-glucan). In 1984, a patent was issued in Japan to Nanba and others.

Maitake has been used in Japan to treat diabetes and high blood pressure and is also known to lower blood cholesterol. But it is the anti-cancer properties that chiefly interest us. Recently, a team of scientists from the department of urology at New York Medical College, in Valhalla, conducted experiments on the effect of maitake on prostate cancer cells. The scientists isolated and grew hormone-resistant prostate cancer cells, and then treated the cells with a highly purified beta-glucan extract from maitake (Grifon-D). After 24 hours of incubation, nearly all the cancer cells had died. The same team also found that vitamin C has a synergistic effect with Grifon-D. They concluded that vitamin C and maitake in combination have antioxidant effects (antioxidants help reverse the damage that free radicals do to body tissue). This combination may be useful as an alternative therapy for prostate cancer.

Researchers at Gunma University, in Japan, conducted an experiment to determine the inhibiting effect of different mushroom extracts on bladder cancer. For the experiment, laboratory mice were fed a carcinogen called BBN, which is known to cause cancer of the bladder. The mice were divided into four groups: one group was given no mushroom extracts, while the other three groups were given either shiitake mushrooms, maitake mushrooms, or Pleurotus ostreatus (oyster mushrooms). After eight weeks, all the mice in the group that received no mushroom extracts had contracted bladder cancer. In the maitake group, 46.7 percent had contracted cancer compared to 52.9 percent in the shiitake group and 65 percent in the oyster mushroom group.

The experiment also yielded interesting results concerning macrophages. Macrophages are attracted to cells that appear to be foreign. Carcinogens such as BBN, however, suppress macrophages' ability to find foreign cells quickly. This experiment revealed that mushrooms protected the macrophages' ability from being affected by BBN. The three mushrooms also had similar effects on lymphocytes, the white cells that circulate in the lymph and flush viruses and other pathogens from the body. Lymphocyte activity in the control group of mice was impaired, while the mice in the mushroom groups remained normal.

Nanba's group also reported preliminary date on maitake's use as an adjunct to chemotherapy in 1997. A non-randomized clinical trial using maitake D-fraction was conducted. There were a total of 165 patients, 25–65 years old, with stage III or IV cancer. The results suggested that patients with cancer of the breast, lung, or liver were improved. Some of the chemotherapy side effects, such as loss of appetite, vomiting, nausea, and hair loss, were ameliorated.

Researchers have known for some time that 1-3 and 1-6 beta-glucans aid the immune system and that beta-glucans from different mushrooms aid the immune system in different ways. Maitake, for example, stimulates macrophages to produce more cytokines (chemical messengers that alert the immune system). Scientists from the Tokyo University of Pharmacy and Life Science conducted experiments on a cytokine called tumor necrosis factor alpha (TNF-()). This toxin-like substance is especially adept at killing malignant tumor cells. The scientists found that macrophages release TNF-(after they have taken up certain types of high–molecular weight beta-glucans found in maitake. Another study at Tokyo College of Pharmacy found that maitake stimulated the production of another cytokine, interleukin-6 (IL-6), which is important in the defense against tumor cells. Researchers at Kobe Pharmaceutical University also found that the maitake D-fraction activates macrophages, dendritic cells, and T cells, enhances the cytotoxicity of natural killer (NK) cells through the production of interleukin-12 (IL-12), and in general confirmed the activity of the beta-glucans of *Grifola frondosa* on diverse parts of our immune defenses against cancer.

SHIITAKE

In the 1960s, Japanese researchers undertook a series of epidemiological studies to learn everything they could about incidences of disease in their country. In one study, they found two remote mountain villages where cancer was nearly unheard of. The government sent teams of scientists to these villages to ascertain why cancer rates were so low there. Was it something about how the people lived? Was it something in the diet? It so happened that growing shiitake mushrooms was the chief industry in both places and the inhabitants ate a lot of shiitake.

The name *shiitake* comes from the Japanese word for a variety of chestnut tree, *shita,* and the word for mushroom, *take.* Shiitake is sometimes called the forest mushroom. In China, it is known as *shaingugu,* which means "fragrant mushroom." Another name is *Hua gu,* which means "white flower mushroom," referring to the cracked white "donko" variety of shiitake. Shiitake's Latin name is *Lentinula edodes.*

After the white button mushroom (*Agaricus bisporus*), shiitake is the most popular culinary mushroom in the world. The cultivation of shiitake in the United States is increasing faster than the cultivation of any other culinary mushroom. Shiitake's meaty flavor can complement almost any dish and, as it turns out, the mushroom that delights so many with its distinctive flavor is also a medicinal mushroom. Even among mushrooms, shiitake is high in nutrition: it contains all the essential amino acids, as well as eritadenine, a unique amino acid that some physicians believe lowers cholesterol. Shiitake is also high in iron, niacin, and B vitamins, especially B1 and B2. In sun-dried form, it contains vitamin D. Hot water extracts from cultured mycelium of *Lentinula edodes* contain polysaccharide KS-2 and a peptide containing the amino acids serine, threonine, alanine, and proline.

The shiitake mushroom is native to Japan, China, Korea, and other areas of East Asia. The cap is dark brown at first and grows lighter with age. The spores are white and the edges of the gills are serrated. In the wild, shiitake grows on dead or dying hardwood trees (chestnut, beech, oak, Japanese alder, mulberry, and others) during the winter and spring. It prefers forest shade where cold water is nearby. The shiitake industry in Japan, as large as it is, can be credited with preserving much of the nation's forests. Without income from shiitake, many a yeoman farmer would have long ago cut down his trees or sold his land to developers. Shiitake mushrooms are Japan's leading agricultural export. Japan used to account for 80 percent of worldwide shiitake production, but China exports considerably more than Japan now. The city of Qingyuan is said to produce more than half of the world's shiitake crop.

Shiitake cultivation in the United States got off to a slow start. For much of the last century, the U.S. Department of Agriculture (USDA) imposed a complete quarantine on the importation of shiitake mushrooms, because they mistook it for another mushroom with a similar sounding name, *Lentinus lepideus*. This mushroom, also called "Train Wrecker," was known to attack and corrode railroad ties and was the suspect in several railway mishaps. In 1972, the USDA realized its mistake and lifted the quarantine against shiitake. Today, American growers produce approximately five million pounds (2.2 tons) of shiitake annually.

In nature, the shiitake fungus propagates and spreads from spores produced by the mushroom. However, for cultivation, spore germination is too unreliable. Instead, logs are inoculated with actively growing fungus. The fungus is first adapted to wood by growing it directly on small pieces of wood. Active fungal cultures intended as inoculum for mushroom cultivation are called spawn. Because the quality of the crop can be no better than the spawn, growers must use viable shiitake spawn of a good variety in pure culture, free of weed fungi and bacteria.

In China, the cultivation of shiitake mushrooms began about 1,000 years ago with a woodcutter named Wu San-kwung in the mountainous regions of Zhejiang province. To test his axe, he swung it against a fallen log on which shiitake mushrooms grew. Days later he noticed shiitake mushrooms growing where his axe landed. On one occasion, the story goes, mushrooms failed to grow on a log and he grew frustrated. He attacked the log vigorously with the blade of his axe. When he returned next to the scene, he discovered that the battered log was full of mushrooms. In this way the "soak and strike" method of cultivation was found, in which logs are battered in such a way as to allow the spores more openings to germinate. Wu San-kwung's contributions to agriculture are commemorated in a temple in Qingyuan and festivals in his name are still celebrated throughout Zhejiang province.

Immunomodulating activities of *Lentinula edodes* extracts decrease rapidly when the mushrooms have been stored at 20°C for seven days, while no decrease occurs at low temperature storage (between 1°C and 5°C). It is imperative that medicinal mushrooms be harvested when they contain the optimum beta-glucan concentration and that the harvested fruit bodies should be stored at the correct temperature before processing or consumption. Drying stops the beta-glucan loss.

In 1969, Tetsuro Ikekawa of Purdue University, working in conjunction with researchers at the National Cancer Center Research Institute, in Tokyo, extracted a 1-3 beta-glucan from shiitake that he tested in mice infected with tumors. Tumor growth was inhibited in 72 to 92 percent of the animals. From this study, the drug Lentinan was developed. By 1976, scientists had completed clinical trials and developed a pharmaceutical version of the drug. The Japanese government's Health and Welfare Ministry approved the drug. However, although this is the Japanese equivalent to Food and Drug Administration approval in the United States, approval in other countries did not occur and the drug is only available in Japan.

Lentinan is used extensively in Japan to treat a variety of tumors. Interestingly, it does not have direct anti-cancer activity—when the drug is incubated in the test tube with tumor cells, cell killing does not occur. However, when given to cancer patients, the drug leads to production of anti-tumor T cells and natural killer cells. It is the third most widely prescribed anti-cancer drug in the world and has an excellent safety profile through many years of use in Japan.

7

New Beginnings

iological therapy is a new approach to cancer treatment that may be used alongside the traditional methods of surgery, radiation, and chemotherapy. Biological therapy consists of the use of living cells given directly to patients or of cellular products such as growth factors that can be produced in standardized forms using biotechnology. This has developed into a large field of science, technology, and medicine.

EARLY EXAMPLES OF BIOLOGICAL AGENTS

Some relatively non-specific biological agents have been available for more than half a century. These early examples of biological drugs are not highly targeted and, in some cases, their actions are even now not precisely understood, although it is obvious that they act via the immune system.

Bacillus Calmette-Guérin (BCG)

One of the first such drugs to be used is known as bacillus Calmette-Guérin (BCG). BCG was originally developed as a vaccine against tuberculosis. This agent is a powerful immune adjuvant, a substance that non-specifically enhances the immune response to an antigen. Today, BCG continues to play an important role in the immune therapy of bladder cancer, with many thousands of patients treated every year, despite the fact that the precise mechanisms of action are still not understood. This relatively uncomplicated approach of instilling a live culture of the bacterium into the bladder is arguably one of the most successful examples of harnessing immune responses to treat cancer.

Bladder cancer is the fourth most common cancer among men and the eighth most common among women in the developed world, with 54,000 new cases occurring annually in the United States, and 11,000 people dying of the disease. A similar picture is observed in the European Union, with the highest incidences in Denmark, Belgium, Italy, and the United Kingdom. Superficial bladder cancer can be treated surgically, whereas highly advanced disease requires chemotherapy, albeit with a high risk for toxicity associated with this treatment. In between these two extremes are many patients who can be treated with BCG. A recent British report showed that BCG produced a response rate of between 50 and 60 percent for papillary tumors and between 70 and 80 percent for carcinoma *in situ* (a very early stage of cancer). These good clinical responses are sustained with remissions averaging 70 percent for five years. BCG is significantly less toxic than chemo- therapy and is very well tolerated by most patients. BCG produces greater benefit for preventing recurrence than chemotherapy (14 percent versus 44 percent in a British report), at least for early cancers.

Interferons

Another early example of a biological drug are the interferons. In 1957, researchers discovered the phenomenon of viral interference—that infection by viruses induced the body of the host to produce factors that inhibit or interfere with the growth and infective ability of other viruses and chemical factors. They named the new factors "interferons." Interferons are among the first of a new class of biological agents called cytokines, which are essentially messengers that allow cells to communicate with each other. Since the discovery of interferon, many additional cytokines have been found and some have become useful in cell therapy. Scientists have described two main types of interferon: type I, of which the most important member is interferon-(, and type II, of which includes interferon-(. Interferon-(is secreted by T cells and is part of the powerful cell-based anti-cancer response, but both types are useful in cancer treatment.

In the 1970s, the Wellcome Foundation, in the United Kingdom, began production of interferon-(with a cell culture technology for clinical use. Today, however, it is made using genetic engineering by inserting the cloned interferon gene into bacteria and growing the bacteria in large bioreactors. Interferon-(has been found to be useful for the treatment of chronic myeloid leukemia (CML), multiple myeloma, and other blood cancers, but its use has to some extent been replaced in these diseases by newer drugs. It is still widely used in the treatment of kidney cancer and melanoma, a highly malignant form of skin cancer, sometimes in combination with other immune therapies.

Interleukin-2 (IL-2)

An important biological drug available in a highly standardized form is the cytokine interleukin-2 (IL-2). IL-2 stimulates the growth of T cells, which are cells of the immune system that can mount powerful defenses against cancer. During the 1970s, many such messenger molecules were discovered and initially confusing names were given to them, some with wildly optimistic connotations, such as leukemia inhibitory factor. A respected committee of scientists was then formed and created the new terminology of interleukins (meaning "between white cells"), with the prefix IL. Currently, there are more than 30 recognized ILs, many available in a standardized form produced using genetic engineering technology. Some are used predominantly in the laboratory and some have shown promise as gene therapy, while others are given to patients as biological drugs.

Clinically, IL-2 is the most important cytokine discovered to date. From the early 1970s onward, Steven Rosenberg and colleagues at the National Cancer Institute pioneered the use of IL-2, either alone or with other biological modalities or chemotherapy, for the treatment of kidney cancer and melanoma—two types of cancer that used to be fatal when occurring at an advanced stage. These researchers achieved a first in biological therapy, the complete cure of a small but significant proportion of patients. Not only did the cancer completely disappear in response to IL-2 treatment in some patients, but also, and most strikingly, the cancer never returned in many of these patients (complete remissions). In a long-term report, published in 1999, 60 percent of patients with melanoma who had complete remissions remained free of disease up to eight years later. The response for patients with kidney cancer was even more striking, with 80 percent of complete responses maintained in the long term. Admittedly, only a minority of patients (less than 10 percent) achieved this complete response, which is the prerequisite for cure. Even so, the long-term cure of patients with widespread disease was a genuine triumph for biological therapy and stimulated the search for further advances.

IL-2 was also found to improve the results for bone marrow transplant recipients with several types of leukemia and lymphoma. However, these highly promising results had significant associated problems, with many patients developing a complication called capillary leak syndrome, which had to be treated in intensive care units. Eventually, with further fine-tuning of the method of administration, these problems could be managed. Today, administration of the drug is by injection of relatively small doses under the skin, sometimes together with interferon, and the treatment can be done on an outpatient basis with relatively few side effects. Tens of thousands of patients have now been treated with IL-2-based therapies.

Other interleukins found applications in the laboratory development of cellular immune therapy, enabling researchers to switch on and off cell receptors and to culture large numbers of desired cells. These include IL-1, IL-4, IL-6, and a related cytokine called tumor necrosis factor (TNF). All are available as genetically engineered products, thus greatly increasing the scope for laboratory scientists.

Colony-Stimulating Factors (CSFs)

Another large family of biological messengers are blood cell growth factors called colony-stimulating factors (CSFs), which stimulate the growth of cell colonies on culture plates in controlled laboratory conditions. CSFs are also cytokines because they mediate movement or action between different types of cells through receptors on the cell surface.

Erythropoietin (EPO), the first CSF developed, is a true hormone and stimulates the growth of red blood cells by the bone marrow. It is an important drug for patients undergoing kidney dialysis, who would otherwise have severe anemia. It is widely used to treat the anemia associated with cancer, in many cases improving the quality of life of patients. Two other colony-stimulating factors are widely used today.

Granulocyte colony-stimulating factor (G-CSF) is used to stimulate peripheral blood progenitor cells for use in transplantation. It is also used to increase the number of white blood cells during cancer therapy, often permitting more intensive drug dosages to be given. The second commonly used CSF is granulocyte-macrophage colony-stimulating factor (GM-CSF), which is used in cellular immune therapy for directing the growth and maturation of immune cells such as dendritic cells. The use of these factors has transformed high-dose chemotherapy and bone marrow transplantation, as well as immune therapy.

NEW BIOLOGICAL AGENTS

Due to the enormous expansion in our understanding of cellular biology and genetics, we now have a firm grounding of the molecular basis of disease and, concomitantly, a new approach to medicine based on the strategy of directly targeting the genes and proteins that are pivotal to the development of cancer. Among the first of this new class of biological agents are antibodies that directly target cancer cells or target other molecules such as growth factors for blood vessels, which are important for the growth of tumors. The U.S. Food and Drug Administration (FDA) and similar agencies in Europe and Japan have approved several therapeutic antibodies and more are being developed. The first three approved antibodies are Rituxan(r) (rituximab) for lymphatic cancer, Herceptin(r) (trastuzumab) for breast cancer, and Campath(r) (alemtuzumab) for a type of leukemia. Other are Avastin(r) (bevacizum-ab), which targets the blood vessel growth factor VEGF, Erbitux(r) (cetuximab), which targets the growth factor receptor EGFR, and two that target CD20 (the same receptor molecule targeted by Rituxan) but "armed" with radioactive isotopes—these are Bexxar(r) (tositumomab) and Zevalin(r) (ibritumomab tituxetan). More than ten other monoclonal antibodies are in advanced clinical trials.

Therapeutic antibodies work by homing in on receptors on cell surfaces—for example, breast cancer cells—from a subset of patients expressing the antigen HER2 or the CD20 receptor on lymphoid cells. By the action on these receptors, the result is either turning off the signals within cells (for example, the signals to grow and proliferate) or killing these cells (directly or more usually by natural killer cells and other forms of immune cells). We know that the killing of cancer cells by natural killer cells requires interaction between the Fc-portion of the antibody with receptors supplied by natural killer cells. This process, called antibody-dependent cellular cytotoxicity (ADCC) has been well studied in immunology. In experiments, animals lacking the receptors are resistant to this method of cell kill.

Receptor molecules, such as the HER2 molecule on the surface of breast cancer cells, are trans-membrane receptors, meaning that they have parts that are outside the membrane and parts that are inside. The outside parts (extracellular domains) receive messages and the inside parts (intracellular domains) transmit and amplify the message, often by pairing or otherwise interacting with other domains (this interaction is sometimes referred to as cross-talk). The HER family of trans-membrane receptors are important in amplifying messages that enable cancer cells to grow and divide. By targeting the pivotal molecule HER2, the messages important to the cancer cells can effectively be blocked.

The discovery of monoclonal antibodies has already been described. In the biotechnology industry, this important discovery is a platform that leads to the possibility of producing a virtually unlimited range of biologically useful products to target almost any cellular protein. To briefly summarize, the technique calls for the fusion of an antibody-producing cell and an immortalized malignant cell. The original method described in 1975 produced a mouse antibody. Mouse antibodies are useful for diagnostic methods but it is preferable to have as little mouse protein as possible for clinical use in humans. This is achieved by joining together parts of the antibody molecules of mice (and sometimes rats) and humans to form "chimeric" antibodies, which still have significant mouse sequences, and "humanized" antibodies with limited material from the mice (or rats). Fully human antibodies can now be developed using phage display, a powerful technology for displaying a protein on the surface of a phage (a specific virus) containing the gene that encodes the displayed protein. In this way, antibodies to treat cancer can be custom-made.

Apart from "arming" antibodies by attaching radioactive isotopes or toxins, a number of other strategies to enhance cell kill ability, such as combining antibodies with chemotherapy, are being developed. Bi-specific antibodies, which react with two antigens and can therefore target cancer by bringing an immune killer cell directly to cancer cells, are also being developed. Another promising technique is to attach antibodies to magnetic beads, thus permitting the selection of desired cell populations simply by applying a magnetic field. Both positive selection (selecting desired cells) and negative selection (removing undesired cells) are feasible techniques and are already available in the clinic.

TARGETED THERAPEUTICS

The promise offered by the mapping of the human genome is that whenever we know the precise genetic mechanisms of a given cancer, we can design drugs to target the specific gene or block the action of the protein specified by that gene. A precisely targeted drug of this kind is, of course, the ultimate magic bullet and has been the holy grail of cancer research for many decades. In recent years, apart from the antibodies, several precisely targeted drugs of this type have been developed and approved or are in advanced clinical trials. This represents a giant step forward for the pharmacological approach against cancer, although the diseases these drugs can control with a high rate of success are still relatively rare.

The first molecule to be used in this way was all-trans retinoic acid (ATRA), which is chemically related to vitamin A. In the late 1980s, researchers at Shanghai Second Medical University first discovered that ATRA is useful for the treatment of acute promyelocytic leukemia, inducing complete remissions even in patients previously resistant to treatment. Soon afterwards, researchers in France and the United States confirmed the clinical benefit of ATRA. Chromosome and molecular studies showed that this type of leukemia is caused by a mutation affecting the retinoic acid receptor (RAR) gene, so the action of ATRA has a precise genetic basis. The availability of ATRA has transformed the treatment of this once fatal disease. ATRA has the further advantage of being relatively inexpensive and is given as a tablet by mouth. A specialist experienced in leukemia must still supervise the treatment, as a new type of side effect may be associated with its use, although it is quite manageable. When given with chemotherapy, the long-term outcome for this type of leukemia is excellent. Only a small proportion of patients now require bone marrow transplantation. This advance in the treatment of acute promyelocytic leukemia was followed in recent years by the successful use of arsenic in some cases of this disease. Many clinical teams and research groups report a cure rate of approximately 80 percent.

The second specialized molecular drug to be approved is an inhibitor of a kinase (enzyme) associated with a fused gene called BCR/ABL. This fusion gene is caused by the joining of parts of chromosomes 9 and 22, forming the so-called Philadelphia chromosome. This mutation is the cellular genetic basis of CML and also a minority of cases of acute lymphoblastic leukemia (ALL), especially in adults. The new drug, called imatinib, is more commonly known by its trade name Glivec(r). The discovery of imatinib has been followed by that of dasatinib and nilotinib and indeed a new paradigm in the treatment of CML. These drugs act by blocking various domains of an enzyme specifically produced as a result of the fusion gene BCR/ABL. The development of this new class of drugs has changed the management of these types of leukemia, although bone marrow transplantation is still required for some patients.

Spurred on by these successes, a number of similar targeted approaches are being developed. For example, the drug Iressa(r) (gefitinib) is a specific inhibitor of the enzyme tyrosine kinase of the epidermal growth factor receptor. This drug showed some promise for lung cancer (in Japanese patients with specific gene patterns), although recent data from a clinical trial combining it with chemotherapy showed disappointing results. The epidermal growth factor receptor family is being investigated intensively and more new drugs will no doubt become available in the not too distant future. Since the precise genetic mechanisms for many cancers are not yet known, or may involve a number of genes, this approach will take some time to be available for all cancers.

8

Lingzhi and *Yunzhi*

n Chapter 6, we began our look at medicinal mushrooms and how they are increasingly becoming accepted, both East and West, for their powerful ability to boost the body's own immune defenses. Here, we'll take a closer look at two more species of mushrooms, *lingzhi* (reishi or *Ganoderma lucidum*) and *yunzhi* (*Trametes versicolor*). These mushrooms are commonly used in China, Japan, and elsewhere as an anticancer therapy.

LINGZHI

Lingzhi, also known as reishi, is one of the most revered tonic herbs. The characters "*Ling zhi*" in Chinese mean "spirit plant." It is sometimes called the "ten thousand year mushroom" and the "mushroom of immortality" because of its reputation for promoting longevity. Reishi, the name by which it is often known in the West, comes from the Japanese. The mushroom is also called the "varnished conk" because of its shiny appearance, and the "phantom mushroom" because it is so scarce in the wild. The mushroom's Latin name is *Ganoderma lucidum* (*gan* means "shiny," *derm* means "skin," and *lucidum* means "brilliant").

Reishi has been called the king of herbal medicine, with many herbalists ranking it above ginseng. The late Professor Hiroshi Hikino of the University of Tohoku, in Japan, a premier authority on Eastern medicinal plants, called *lingzhi* "one of the most important elixirs in the Orient." The ancient Chinese text *Shen Nong Ben Jing,* from about AD 500, states that *Ganoderma lucidum* is "useful for enhancing vital energy, increasing thinking faculty, and preventing forgetfulness." It can "refresh the body and mind, delay aging, and enable one to live long. It stabilizes one's mental condition."

In 1995, researchers isolated the DNA of *Ganoderma tsugae* and *Ganoderma lucidum* and found that there were only minor differences between the two species. An even more recent report found that *Ganoderma lucidum* from Asia was in its own group, whereas *Ganoderma lucidum* from Europe and the Americas was more closely related to *Ganoderma tsugae.* Further investigations are needed to resolve the molecular makeup of these species. To make matters even more complicated, there are two different phenotypes: one with the traditional wide shelf-like fruit body and the other antler-shaped and known in Japan as Rokkadu Reishi. The antler form was avidly sought after by ancient Taoists and appears prominently in artwork dating back for centuries. These two types are rumored to have different healing characteristics. Other varieties include *Ganoderma oregonensis* and *Ganoderma applanatum.* All the *Ganoderma* species appear to have essentially the same pharmacologically active compounds.

Lingzhi is not a culinary mushroom. Although some people use the mushroom to brew teas, it is usually taken for medicinal purposes only, as it has a very bitter, woody taste. It contains 119 different triterpenoids, the aromatic substances that have anti-inflammatory, anti-tumor, and antiviral effects. However, the cultured mycelium of the mushroom is not bitter, so people who take it in powder or capsule form need not be bothered by a bitter flavor.

In its natural habitat, the mushroom is found in the dense, humid coastal provinces of China, where it favors the decaying stumps of chestnut, oak, and other broad-leaf trees. In Japan, reishi is usually found on old plum trees. *Lingzhi's* most distinguishing feature is its shiny, lacquered look, which may have contributed to its reputation as an herb that promotes longevity. It has a kidney-shaped cap that does not rot or lose its shape after drying. Sometimes the spores appear on the cap and give the appearance of sandpaper. The mushroom comes in six colors: red (*akashiba*), white (*shiroshiba*), black (*kuroshiba*), blue (*aoshiba*), yellow (*kishiba*) and purple (*murasakishiba*). The red is the one most used for medicinal purposes.

In the wild, these mushrooms are extremely rare and difficult to find. Because the husks of the spores are very hard, the spores cannot germinate as readily as the spores of other mushrooms. Fortunately mycologists are now able to recreate favorable growth conditions. It can be cultured on logs that are buried in shady, moist areas. *Ganoderma lucidum* can also be inoculated into hardwood stumps, and under commercial conditions, it is normally grown on artificial sawdust logs. The herb that was once the provenance of emperors in China can now be purchased from health food stores.

Reishi has a colorful past. According to legend, Taoist priests in the first century were the first to experiment with this mushroom. They included it in magic potions that were supposed to confer longevity and even eternal youth and immortality. These Taoist priests practiced alchemy and were looked upon as magicians or wizards, and by present day standards they might be considered charlatans. But remember, alchemy was the beginning of chemistry, and shamans who treated the sick by summoning the forces of nature to the aid of their patients were the first doctors. A poem by the first century philosopher Wang Chung remarked on the Taoist priests' use of mushrooms in their quest to attain a higher state of consciousness:

> *They dose themselves with the germ of gold and jade*
> *And eat the finest fruit of the purple polypore fungu*
> *By eating what is germinal, their bodies are lightened*
> *And they are capable of spiritual transcendence.*

Ganoderma lucidum achieved pride of place in China's oldest Materia Medica, the *Herbal Classic,* compiled about AD 200. In characteristic Chinese fashion, the *Herbal Classic* divided the 365 herbs that it described into three grades: superior, average, and fair. In the superior grade, *lingzhi* is given first place, ahead of ginseng. To qualify for the superior grade, an herb must have potent medicinal qualities and also produce no ill effects or side effects when taken over a long period of time. The book says of *lingzhi:*

The taste is bitter, its atmospheric energy is neutral; it has no toxicity. It cures the accumulation of pathogens in the chest. It is good for the *chi* of the head, including mental activities. It tonifies the spleen, increases wisdom, and improves memory. Long-term consumption will lighten your body; you will never become old. It lengthens years. It has spiritual power and you will become a spirit being like the immortals.

Lingzhi's reputation as the "mushroom of immortality" reached the Emperor of the Chin dynasty, who was supposed to have outfitted a fleet of ships with a crew of 300 strong men and 300 beautiful women to sail to the East in search of the mushroom. The ships never returned. Legend has it that the shipwrecked castaways washed ashore and founded a new country—Japan.

Lingzhi has been used extensively in China, Korea, and Japan to ameliorate the side effects of radiation therapy. Cancer patients receiving radiation therapy to kill cancer cells frequently experience a reduction of the white blood cells (WBCs), since the radiation damages the bone marrow's ability to produce WBCs, which are necessary to fight infection. It has been shown both in animals and in humans that *lingzhi* can prevent the drastic decrease in WBCs due to radiation.

To examine the immune modulating effects of *lingzhi,* scientists in Taiwan isolated polysaccharides from the fruit-bodies of the mushroom and tested them in the laboratory. They found an increase in three important cytokines, which are molecules secreted by WBCs during an immune response. These cytokines include tumor necrosis factor alpha (TNF-()), interleukin 1-beta (IL-1()), and interleukin 6 (IL-6). These messenger-like factors are important in fighting cancer.

Dr. Hsien-yeh Hsu at the Institute of Biotechnology in Medicine, National Yang-Ming University of Taiwan, and other researchers at the Institute of Biological Chemistry and Genomics Research Center carried out extensive research on *lingzhi* and found polysaccharides that stimulate cytokine production. Their studies show that various immune cells such as macrophages, T and B cells, and natural killer cells are stimulated to kill tumor cells.

Lingzhi also inhibits angiogenesis, the development and growth of blood vessels. Tumors need new blood vessels, otherwise they shrink and die. Scientists found that lingzhi inhibits this process in prostate cancer. Other studies on bladder cancer and breast cancer also showed inhibition of malignant cell growth.

YUNZHI

Trametes versicolor has the distinction of being the mushroom from which one of the world's leading anticancer drugs, Krestin, is derived. Although not been approved by the U.S. Food and Drug Administration, Krestin was the most prescribed anti-cancer drug in Japan for much of the 1980s and 1990s. Approved by Japan's Health and Welfare Ministry, its cost is covered by most health plans in Japan. (A version of *Trametes versicolor* extract, developed by the Chinese University of Hong Kong and made under good manufacturing practices (GMP) in China, is commercially available under the name Oncozac, which contains absorbable peptidoglucans that have been shown to improve immune function.)

In Latin, *Trametes* means "one who is thin" and *versicolor* means "variously coloured." In some literature, the mushroom is called *Coriolus versicolor* or, rarely, *Polyporus versicolor*. In China, the mushroom is called *yunzhi,* which means "cloud mushroom." In Japan, it is called *Kawaratake,* which means "beside-the-river mush-room." In the English-speaking world, the mushroom is known as the "turkey tail" because its fan shape resembles the tail of a standing turkey.

Trametes versicolor is found in temperate forests throughout the world and in all the states of the continental United States. It has a lovely appearance and is occasionally included in floral displays. It is striped with dark and light brown bands that alternate with bands of orange, blue, white, and tan. It prefers to grow on dead logs and has been known to feed on most kinds of trees.

The Japanese have long used this mushroom as a folk remedy for cancer. In traditional Chinese medicine, *yunzhi* is used to treat lung diseases and cancer. Taoists believed that *yunzhi* collected the *yang* energy from the roots of the pine trees where the fungus was commonly found, and they prescribed it for patients whose *yang* energy was deficient.

Trametes versicolor came to the attention of the pharmaceutical industry in 1965, when a chemical engineer working for Kureha Chemical Industry Company, in Japan, observed his neighbor attempting to cure himself of gastric cancer with a folk remedy. The neighbor was in the late stages of cancer and had been rejected for treatment by hospitals and clinics. For several months, he took the folk remedy and then was able to return to work. The folk remedy was *Trametes versicolor*. The engineer convinced his colleagues to examine the mushroom. The best strains of *Trametes versicolor* were found and cultivated. Soon, PSK, an extract from the mushroom, was isolated. PSK is the chief ingredient in Krestin: it is a 1-3 beta-glucan, the type of polysaccharide found in many medicinal mushrooms, but it is bound to a protein and is especially beneficial to the immune system.

The success of Krestin inspired Chinese researchers to develop a *Trametes versicolor* extract of their own called PSP. Both PSK and PSP are potent immune stimulators with specific activity for T cells and for antigen-presenting cells such as macrophages. The biological activity of both is characterized by the ability to increase white blood cell counts and stimulate the production of interferon-(and interleukin-2 (IL-2). Many clinical experiments have been carried out with PSK since 1978 and with PSP since the early 1990s.

PSK is extracted from the mycelia of the strain CM-101 and is approximately 62 percent polysaccharide and 38 percent protein. The glucan portion of PSK consists of a beta 1-4 main chain and beta 1-3 side-chain, with some beta 1-6 chains. After intra-tumoral injection, PSK causes local inflammatory responses that result in the nonspecific killing of the tumor cells. It has been reported that PSK induces gene expression of some cytokines such as TNF-(, IL-1, IL-6, and IL-8. These cytokines, produced by macrophages, monocytes, and various other cell types, directly stimulate cytotoxic T cells against tumors, enhance antibody production by B lymphocytes, and induce IL-2 receptor expression on T cells. The drug is almost always prescribed to cancer patients who have undergone surgery and are undergoing chemotherapy or radiotherapy. It is often prescribed for colon, lung, stomach, and esophageal cancers and has no known side effects. Over 1,000 cancer patients have been treated with Krestin in Japan under a clinical trial setting.

PSP was first isolated from cultured deep-layer mycelium of the COV-1 strain of *Trametes versicolor* in 1983. PSP may contain at least four discrete molecules, all of which are true proteoglycans. PSP differs from PSK in its saccharide makeup—the polysaccharide chains are true beta-glucans. PSP can be easily delivered by the oral route. PSP is prescribed to cancer patients to help improve their immune system before and after surgery, chemotherapy, and radiotherapy. China's Ministry of Public Health approved PSP as a national class I medical material in 1992. In 1999, PSP was added to the list of medicines whose cost could be reimbursed by medical insurance programs in China. The U.S. National Cancer Institute has declared PSP a fungous anticancer substance.

Studies at the University of Shanghai addressed over 650 cancer patients who were undergoing chemotherapy or radiotherapy and concluded that PSP ameliorated many of the side effects of these therapies. PSP has also been found to be synergistic with IL-2 in a number of tumors. Importantly, PSP has been found consistently to ameliorate the bone marrow suppressive effects of chemotherapy. In a double blind, placebo-controlled trial at the Queen Mary Hospital of the University of Hong Kong, the effect of a 28-day administration of PSP for patients completing conventional treatment for advanced non–small cell lung cancer was evaluated. There was a significant improvement in the WBCs and antibody response in the treated group. In another study, PSP was found to stimulate lymphokine-activated killer cells (LAK cells) and reduce the concentration of IL-2 needed to produce a cytotoxic response. PSP was also found to be very safe, with no evidence of toxic effects in animal studies or in human clinical trials.

9

Invaders
and Defenders

recent focus of cancer research is the development of cancer vaccines. Most of us are familiar with the idea of vaccination for measles, polio, and other infectious diseases. In these cases, vaccines seek to activate an immune response—put the immune system on active duty, so to speak—by exposing it to a non-infective version of the organism. At this time, cancer vaccines remain mostly experimental, but scientists believe a similarly powerful activation of the immune response can be accomplished for cancer.

THE DISCOVERY OF VACCINATION

In the modern sense, vaccination refers to the deliberate introduction of an antigen into the body to elicit a specific immune response. The discovery of vaccination is a wonderful story of how astute observation combined with deductive logic can launch a revolution in health care affecting the lives of millions of people.

Edward Jenner (1749–1823) was a vicar's son who became a pupil of the eminent surgeon John Hunter. Hunter was an amateur scientist, basing his studies on observations of natural phenomena. As a surgeon, Jenner could have had a successful practice in London, but chose to return to Gloucester in the English countryside. At that time, smallpox was a much-feared disease not dissimilar to the situation with cancer today, with a high mortality rate and life-long disfigurement of survivors. However, it was known that if you survived the acute illness, then you became immune to subsequent exposure. In the countryside, Jenner became aware that some people developed a much milder pox-like illness known as cowpox, which is endemic among cattle, and subsequently became immune to smallpox. Jenner collected a series of ten such people. In 1796, he took some lymph from the finger of a dairymaid who was suffering from cowpox and inoculated the material into a healthy boy. Six weeks later, the boy was exposed to smallpox but did not develop the disease. Jenner then went on to produce dried vaccine from the cowpox virus, variola. This epoch-defining achievement became universally accepted and vaccination against smallpox was made compulsory in Britain in 1853. The British government awarded Jenner a sum of 30,000 pounds, a huge fortune in the eighteenth century, and Napoleon had his army vaccinated.

Another pioneer of vaccination was the French scientist Louis Pasteur, one of the most talented innovators of all time, with great powers of intuition as well as logical deduction. Pasteur initially worked with silkworms and only succeeded in preventing an illness in a larger animal model relatively late in his life—in this case, chicken-cholera. In 1879, by a fortuitous chance, he noted that if a chicken-cholera bacillus culture was "aged," it became attenuated and failed to produce the disease if inoculated into chickens. Nevertheless, the inoculated chickens became resistant on exposure to fresh culture. Pasteur also made a vaccine against anthrax and staged a successful demonstration at an agricultural exhibition in 1881. Pasteur went on to make his famous discovery of the rabies vaccine. In 1885, he cured nine-year-old Joseph Meister, who had been bitten fourteen times by a rabid dog. The child survived and later became a caretaker at the Pasteur Institute. In 1886, Pasteur's method was used to treat 2,671 patients and only 25 died. Today, his studies are considered classical examples of clinical trials.

THE VACCINE PARADIGM AND CANCER

How can this classical paradigm of utilizing immune responses to prevent or treat disease be applied to cancer? We have previously noted that modern immunology has unveiled mechanisms in the

host defense against cancer. Cancer vaccines and cellular immunotherapy for cancer in general are based on the simple premise that
there are fundamentally only two types of cells involved in cancer—invaders and defenders. Cancer cells are the invading cells
and the outcome of the body's struggle against cancer may in large
measure depend on its defenders, the cells of the immune system.

Until recently, scientists thought that the immune system constantly patrolled for cancer cells, actively preventing cancer. Cancer, therefore, appeared to be a result of a failure of surveillance.
We now know that this is too simplistic. To maintain health, the
immune system must be able to tolerate large numbers of antigens, including many that are not of host origin but which nevertheless are not dangerous. An important problem is that in
some cases, perhaps even the majority, the dendritic cells (white
blood cells that typically use threadlike tentacles to enmesh antigen, which they present to T cells) do not recognize cancer antigens as posing a danger in the same way that viruses are
recognized. This could be because viral infection causes inflammation and necrosis, a form of violent cell death, whereas in cancer there is no such signal.

From this, it becomes clear that there is a difference between
vaccination against a viral disease such as measles and vaccination
against cancer. In the case of measles, we are dealing with people
who have not yet been exposed to the measles virus. By simply
exposing them to a modified, less virulent form of the virus, the
dendritic cells sense the danger signals and present the antigen for
an activation response and everything proceeds in the expected
manner. In contrast, for the patient with cancer, there has already
been exposure to an antigen but the danger signal is not given or
the co-stimulation molecules are not expressed. Therefore, in cancer, the challenge is to present the antigen in a form that does not
result in tolerance.

There are many approaches to the development of cancer vaccines. From the standpoint of the pharmaceutical industry, it is
obviously desirable to develop standardized "off-the-shelf" vaccines that could be based on defined antigens or the DNA that
specifies these antigens. This approach would lead to the mass production, for example, of vials of vaccines as drugs for a given type

of cancer. However, with the possible exception of vaccines against melanoma, this approach has been unsuccessful to date, although intensive effort is ongoing.

In the 1980s and 1990s, approaches using the cancer cells of the patient being treated as the source of vaccines proved more successful. These are called autologous vaccines (derived from the same individual) and are the simplest way to produce a cancer vaccine. The use of autologous tumor cells overcomes many of the difficulties associated with the need to present an antigen within the framework of the major histocompatibility complex (MHC), a system that defines "self" and "non-self" and is important in the transplant context. A large number of pre-clinical and clinical studies have reported using this approach to treat a variety of human cancers, including cancers of the lung, breast, ovary, and kidney, as well as melanoma.

Early-stage colon cancer has been the subject of two randomized controlled clinical trials using autologous vaccines, with long periods of follow-up. In an American study, published in the *Journal of Clinical Oncology* in 1993, patients with colon and rectal cancer with a significant risk of relapse were randomly treated with either surgery alone or surgery followed by autologous vaccination; radiation therapy was also given for patients with rectal cancer. The results showed that, for colon cancer, the recurrence rate for vaccinated patients after 6.5 years was 25 percent compared to 56.5 percent for the control group, who did not receive vaccinations. The mortality rate for patients receiving vaccination was 16.7 percent compared with 47.8 percent for the control patients. However, this study has been criticized for technical and statistical flaws. Only a proportion of patients had adequate vaccination as judged by skin tests. There were a relatively small numbers of patients enrolled in the study and the results did not reach statistical significance. Also, patients with rectal cancer did not enjoy clinical benefit, a result that the researchers attributed to the use of radiation soon after vaccination. So, although the report generated much interest, it was regarded as preliminary only and subject to confirmation.

More definitive results were obtained in another phase III randomized, controlled trial carried out in Europe by the Dutch

Clinical Trials with Human Subjects

In 1961, the eighteenth World Medical Assembly, recognizing that medical progress is based on research, which ultimately must encompass experimentation involving human subjects, adopted the Declaration of Helsinki. This protocol has been revised and updated at subsequent meetings of the Assembly and is widely accepted as setting forth the required ethical standards for experimental treatments.

To facilitate international collaboration in clinical trials, the regulatory bodies of the European Union, the United States, and Japan established a common mechanism known as the International Conference on Harmonization (ICH). The ICH established guidelines for Good Clinical Practice (GCP), which form the standards for the conduct of clinical trials. Important elements of GCP include the establishment of institutional review boards or ethics committees and the detailed explanations that must be given to clinical trial subjects for informed consent.

• A phase I clinical trial is one in which the objective is to find out how the human body reacts to a new drug or experimental treatment being investigated—for example, the appropriate dose and whether or not there is any toxicity. Because the drug or treatment being tested may be completely new, it is also necessary to determine the optimal route of administration and dosing schedule. The expected efficacy is a secondary concern at this stage.

• In a phase II clinical trial, the objective is to find out whether there is any efficacy. Patients in a phase II trial frequently have advanced disease or have already failed treatment with a number of available drugs.

• In a phase III clinical trial, the test treatment is compared with the standard treatment (control) for a particular disease. This is usually done by randomly assigning patients to the standard or to the experimental treatments.

Clinical trials are frequently designed and operated by independent clinical research organizations (CROs). In general, clinical research for cell therapy, such as cell-based cancer vaccines, follows the format for clinical trials of drugs, although additional guidelines for good tissue practice (GTP) have been developed. There are also standards for clinical manufacturing facilities for the laboratories involved in cellular therapy.

National Cancer Institute and published in the *Lancet* in 1999. This study included 254 patients with colon cancer treated with surgery alone or surgery followed by autologous tumor cell vaccination. For the vaccinated group, there was a 41 percent reduction in the risk of recurrence after a median follow-up of 5.3 years. However, this benefit appeared to be restricted to those patients with stage II colon cancer. For this subset of patients who received the vaccine, as compared to those who did not, the risk reduction was 61 percent, a highly significant outcome.

Both these studies utilized cancer cells obtained at the time of surgery and made into single cell suspensions, which were then irradiated to prevent growth of the malignant cells. The production of vaccine is relatively straightforward and involves using an enzyme to process the solid pieces of tumor. A degree of technical skill is critical, since excess enzyme may damage cell surface antigens needed for the vaccine to work. The irradiated cells are stored frozen. When required for use, the cell suspension is thawed and then mixed with an immune adjuvant to enhance the response. Both the immune adjuvant BCG (bacillus Calmette-Guérin) and the growth factor GM-CSF (granulocyte-macrophage colony-stimulating factor) can be used in this setting. No other significant side effects have been reported using this simple and inexpensive technique.

DENDRITIC CELL–BASED IMMUNE THERAPY

By the early 1990s, it was clear to most researchers in the field that the relatively straightforward approach described above for autologous vaccines may have efficacy for early-stage colon cancer. A similar vaccine has also been reported to be successful in preventing tumor recurrence in early-stage kidney cancer. However, it also became clear that for clinical situations involving more advanced cancer, a more powerful vaccine was desirable.

Much has now been learned about dendritic cells, which account for less than one percent of the white blood cells in the peripheral circulation. The first successful culture of human dendritic cells was reported in 1992, but it was not until two years later that a breakthrough occurred. This was the development of a relatively simple method of generating large numbers of dendritic cells from white blood cells by culture with the cytokines interleukin 4 (IL-4) and GM-CSF. Further research into the use of proinflammatory cytokines, such as IL-1, IL-6, and tumor necrosis factor (TNF)-(, as maturation stimuli led to reliable methods of producing dendritic cells ex-vivo, which have become widely used in immune therapy strategies. Many laboratories can now routinely generate dendritic cells for vaccine therapy.

Dendritic cell–based immune therapy was successfully tested in animal models. In 2004, Gunnar Kvalheim, a leading Norwegian researcher, summarized the state of the art of dendritic cell vaccines. More than 500 patients had been treated in over 30 clinical trials using different protocols. The overall response rate was around 20 percent, with occasional complete responses and many patients having prolonged stable disease. These patients have good quality of life, although their cancer has not been eradicated. However, the current results need improvement and a number of new strategies, both clinical and in the laboratory, are being innovated.

The biotechnology company Dendreon has adopted the cellular drug strategy and has several products in the pipeline. One is a dendritic cell vaccine for prostate cancer called Provenge(r), which has completed phase III clinical trials. In March 2007, the U.S. Food and Drug Administration (FDA) approved this "cellular drug," making it the first therapeutic cancer vaccine to be so approved. Provenge is custom-made for the individual patient, who must have his or her white blood cells collected using a cell separator. This could be done, for example, in blood transfusion centers or at a cancer clinic. A designated courier then transports the collected cells to the company's central processing facility, where the cells are cultured and the dendritic cells are harvested. A patented molecule, based on an antigen on the surface of prostate cancer cells fused with the growth factor GM-CSF, is used to process the dendritic cells. The dendritic cells containing the special fusion molecule is then transported back to the clinic and administered to the patient. This is an approach requiring very intensive and costly logistics. The clinical trials show good promise for patients with less aggressive forms of prostate cancer but

Provenge may not be suitable for all patients. Dendreon has two other dendritic cell vaccines in relatively advanced clinical trials, one is based on the breast cancer cellular receptor molecule HER2, the same receptor targeted by the monoclonal antibody trastuzumab, and is preliminarily reported to be active even in patients whose disease is resistant to trastuzumab. The company is also actively testing another product designed for the treatment of myeloma, a form of bone marrow cancer.

In Europe and Asia, many groups favor a less centralized approach to produce a dendritic cell vaccine. They point out the great complexities of transporting individual patients' cells to and from the central manufacturing plant. In Europe and Asia, such transportation of cells would have to cross and re-cross national borders and the logistics would be difficult. There is another consideration: we all want to take pride in our community. For cellular therapy to be truly successful, we must envisage a future in which each community hospital will have a department of "cancer immuno-therapy." But what must be done to promote a decentralized strategy for cancer vaccines and cell therapy in general? One answer is that, like all other human endeavors of a collaborative nature, the importance of a division of labor cannot be overstated. This has been true from the making of Stone Age implements to space exploration.

OTHER CELL-BASED THERAPEUTIC APPROACHES

Natural killer cells (NK cells) have anti-cancer activity and do not require prior activation. An early model of NK-like cells in cancer therapy used lymphokine-activated killer (LAK) cells, discovered by Steven Rosenberg and colleagues at the National Cancer Institute in the 1970s. They developed a method of growing large numbers of LAK cells from lymphocytes collected from the peripheral blood. The cells were grown in culture containing the T-cell growth factor IL-2. Following pre-clinical studies that showed tumor responses in animals, a number of pilot clinical trials and randomized trials involving more than 600 patients compared LAK cells plus IL-2 with IL-2 alone. These studies were mostly done during the 1980s, when IL-2 was available only in limited quantities and therefore not in general use. In a recent summary of 679 patients with advanced kidney cancer treated with LAK cells plus IL-2, the overall response rate was 25 percent, with 8 percent achieving a complete response. Many of the complete responses were durable, meaning that the cancer did not return after many years of follow-up.

Rosenberg's group went on to study tumor-infiltrating lymphocytes (TILs), prepared from tumors obtained at the time of surgery. In certain culture conditions, the tumor cells die off, leaving a pure growth of lymphocytes with anti-cancer properties. These can be further cultured or expanded to very large numbers. TILs are much more powerfully active against cancer than lymphocytes that have never been exposed to cancer. In a recent summary of 115 patients from various research groups, there was a 23.2 percent overall response to the TIL approach, with a complete response rate of 6 percent. Again, many of the complete responses were long-term cures. These studies established that reproducible results, including long-term freedom from cancer in a small subset of patients, could be achieved using a cellular immune therapeutic strategy, even for advanced cancer.

From the perspective of the year 2007, these studies of LAK cells and TILs performed in the 1980s had a number of defects. Research in the 1980s had not yet elucidated the molecular structure of IL-2 receptors, leading to the use of relatively large doses of IL-2 in infusions and cultures. The culture methodology was complex and the entire process highly intensive. However, interest in NK-like cells has recently been revived, with a new understanding of their receptor biology and their possible role in mediating the graft-vs-tumor response. A recent development is that of cytokine-induced killer (CIK) cells, which have active anti-cancer activity and can be produced in large quantities in laboratory systems. NK-like cells are a good source of Fc-(receptors, which could be important for enhancing the action of antibodies through antibody-dependent cellular cytotoxicity (ADCC). Recently, the NK-92 cell line has entered clinical trials in Europe and the United States. Thus, although LAK cells and TILs are no longer used, many useful lessons were learned that are likely to find applications in the future.

"PRIMED" LYMPHOCYTES

Another approach to developing a more powerful response to vaccination is to collect lymphocytes after vaccination and to culture the lymphocytes using the monoclonal antibody to the receptor molecule CD3. The T-cell receptor can be activated using the CD3 antibody. It is then possible to use IL-2 to stimulate T-cell proliferation. In this way, very large numbers of T cells can be generated that can be re-infused into patients for anti-tumor activity and to enhance endogenous immune responses.

Preliminary studies in animals bearing transplanted tumors showed that this combination of vaccination and the culture of primed lymphocytes is a feasible strategy, resulting in immune tumor rejection in the majority of treated animals. In the clinic, the strategy is simple and straightforward. Tumor cells are collected from the patient, either using a biopsy needle or preserved in liquid nitrogen at the time of surgery. The cells are irradiated so that they can no longer multiply but the cancer antigens are still preserved. These irradiated cells can be simply mixed with an adjuvant, such as BCG or GM-CSF, and then injected into sites where there is good lymphatic drainage, such as under the arms and in the groin. After a suitable time and, in many cases, after further vaccinations to enhance the immune response, the activated lymphocytes can be collected. These activated lymphocytes can then be cultured in the laboratory to increase their cell numbers, a process known as ex-vivo expansion. Very large numbers of such cells, up to hundreds of billions, can be grown and re-infused into patients with minimal side effects, to help eradicate cancer cells.

Gary Wood and colleagues applied this strategy to treat nine patients with aggressive brain cancer resistant to surgery, radiation, and chemotherapy. Two of the nine patients are now long-term tumor-free with no maintenance therapy. This is particularly impressive because these patients had terminal cancer and the survival of the non-responders was only 4–6 months. The treatment was well tolerated, with fever during the re-infusion of cells being the main side effect observed.

This approach has been successfully used to treat other types of cancer. Alfred Chang and his group at the University of Michigan, using vaccine primed lymph node cells instead of peripheral blood cells, successfully treated about fifty patients with kidney cancer. They reported responses of up to 40 percent; many of the responding patients have long-term control of their cancer.

What happens if a T-cell strategy is desired but there is no tumor tissue saved from the time of the original surgery and there is no readily available source of autologous tumor cells that can be obtained by biopsy? This is a frequent scenario and the answer might lie in a technology called auto-lymphocyte therapy (ALT), which refers to a cellular strategy based on the activation of memory T cells. For the majority of patients with cancer, the immune system has already been exposed to cancer antigens but developed tolerance or some other avoidance mechanism. We can therefore reason that memory T cells already exist, and so antigen re-exposure by the process of vaccination may not be necessary. In a sense, the patient has already been vaccinated via the exposure to cancer. This is particularly true of patients with metastatic disease. However, in many such patients, the tumor has already developed an avoidance mechanism against the host immune system, perhaps by turning some of the host immune cells (regulatory T cells) against the fighting. Nevertheless, auto-lymphocyte therapy is an interesting concept.

For culturing activated memory T cells, specific cytokines are collected and used to activate a second cohort of cells. ALT has been extensively studied in advanced kidney cancer. In a phase II trial, Krane and colleagues achieved delayed progression of disease in 33 percent of patients. The one-year survival rate was 56 percent and two-year survival was 36 percent in a group of patients with a poor prognosis. In a multi-center phase III study, ALT plus cimetidine (an anti-ulcer drug with activity against immune suppressor cells) was compared to cimetidine alone. Initial studies showed that patients receiving the cellular therapy survived twenty-one months compared with only eight months for the control patients. Updated results continued to show a survival advantage for cellular therapy, leading to its use in the clinical practice setting in Boston, Atlanta, Georgia, and Orange County, California. Patients tolerated the treatment well with virtually no side effects, apart from fever at the time of infusion of activated T cells. However, at the time this book goes to press, ALT is a somewhat neglected approach.

A LINK BETWEEN VIRUSES AND CANCER?

The relationship of viruses to human cancer is one of the most fascinating subjects in cancer research. The core of a virus consists of a relatively short strand of nucleic acid; antigens on the surface or in the core can be easily cloned. Much more detail is known about viruses than cancer cells, at least at the present state of research. What is more, it is already known that some viruses are associated with human cancer. For example, preventing hepatitis B and C by vaccination and improvement in blood transfusion practices can dramatically reduce the incidence of liver cancer. Although the effect of such preventive measures needs many years to be translated into lives definitely saved, recent data from Taiwan show that such reduction in liver cancer through vaccination against hepatitis is no longer in doubt. Another important advance is the recent approval by the FDA of Gardasil, a vaccine against four common types of the human papilloma virus (HPV), which is the cause of genital warts and of cervical cancer. Vaccination against HPV in girls before sexual maturity is likely to lead to a dramatic reduction in cervical cancer.

One of the viruses intensively studied in relation to cancer is the Epstein-Barr virus (EBV), which plays an important role in a number of human diseases. The human species has lived for hundreds of thousands of years with EBV. The diseases associated with EBV include Burkitt lymphoma (a type of lymphoid cancer found in endemic form in some parts of Africa and more rarely in the developed world), Hodgkin's disease, nasopharyngeal carcinoma (very common in China and Southeast Asia), and others. A particularly devastating form of EBV-associated malignancy is an aggressive lymphoma-like illness with a very high mortality rate called EBV-associated lympho-proliferative disease (EBV-LPD), which often strikes patients with a compromised immune system. There is a high rate of EBV-LPD following bone marrow or blood stem cell transplantation, and sometimes in solid organ transplant recipients as well. The story of the successful prevention and treatment of EBV-LPD, particularly in the post-transplant setting, is very dramatic, although so far involves only a relatively small number of patients. This story is undoubtedly a major triumph of cellular immune therapy.

The incidence of EBV-LPD following stem cell transplantation is correlated with the degree of immune suppression. The highest incidence is found among patients receiving partial mismatch-related transplants or unrelated donor transplants. Once EBV-LPD has taken hold, conventional therapy such as chemotherapy is generally ineffective. In 1994, researchers at the Memorial Sloan-Kettering Cancer Center, in New York, reported on the use of unmanipulated donor T cells to treat five patients with EBV-LPD. These researchers based their treatment on the assumption that the donor T cell population would contain cells that are specifically directed at EBV, although the number of such cells would be very small. This was a last attempt at treatment of desperately ill patients. Amazingly, all five patients responded but three developed severe graft-vs-host disease and two patients died of respiratory failure. This report demonstrated that even a very small number of specific T cells could be effective. Presumably these cells underwent large-scale expansion within the body to become a potent anti-tumor force that killed all the EBV-LPD cells. However, the price to be paid in terms of graft-vs-host-related morbidity and mortality is too high for the use of non-selected donor T cells to be routinely recommended.

Malcolm Brenner and co-workers then undertook an extensive program of targeted cellular immune therapy using virus-specific T cells. They established cell lines from more than 120 healthy donors. These cells were infused into patients post–stem cell transplant for the prevention of EBV-LPD. None of the fifty-four patients who received the cells developed EBV-LPD compared with six of fifty-two control patients. This was the first report of successful cellular prophylaxis of a human malignancy. Brenner's group also treated four patients with established EBV-LPD, achieving three complete remissions.

They have now applied a similar strategy to develop cellular therapy for other EBV-associated cancers, such as Hodgkin's disease and nasopharyngeal carcinoma. These are cancers with a relatively high incidence in certain populations. Like EBV-LPD, they express viral antigens, although the pattern of antigen expression is different. Most researchers in this field regard this approach as highly promising and could presage successful therapy in other diseases.

MINI-TRANSPLANTS

We described in previous chapters the use of donor T cells to evoke a powerful graft-vs-tumor response. This has now become routine practice for most transplant teams, either as mini-transplants or as donor lymphocyte infusions for patients who relapse after conventional stem cell transplantation. These graft-vs-tumor responses led to the development of mini-transplant strategies for the treatment of solid tumors. In a mini-transplant, the dose of chemotherapy is relatively light, so that it is well tolerated and can often be given in an outpatient setting. The immune cells of the donor are the main weapons against the cancer cells, as they can recognize the cancer cells through minor transplantation antigens and mount a rejection response. Shimon Slavin who pioneered mini-transplantation, envisages that it can be developed into a platform for the treatment of advanced cancer, provided that the problems of graft-vs-host response can be circumvented. Many groups are working on this approach. One promising strategy, for example, is utilization of NK cells to modulate the graft-vs-host response. A strategy combining vaccination and mini-transplantation has also been successful in a pre-clinical setting, with apparently no graft-vs-host disease. In an update of forty-seven patients with advanced kidney cancer treated with mini-transplants at the National Institutes of Health, there were eighteen partial and four complete responses for a total response rate of 47 percent. Other groups have reported similar encouraging results, including mini-transplants in a small number of cases of breast and ovarian cancer.

10

Winter Worm, Summer Grass

The wonders of *Cordyceps sinensis* have been known in China for at least 1,000 years. It is recognized as a national medicinal treasure, a precious and virtually sacred tonic. As a health supplement, it is known to increase energy and vitality. *Cordyceps* is one of the safest medicinal herbs and is used to treat liver diseases, cancer, heart disease, infertility, and other ailments.

The mushroom has a long and storied past. The first mention of *Cordyceps sinensis* appeared in AD 620 during the Tang dynasty. The literature describes a strange organism that lives high in the mountains of Tibet and is able to change from animal to plant and back to animal again. That sounds far-fetched, but the ancient literature concerning *Cordyceps* is not as bizarre as it seems. *Cordyceps sinensis* is indeed an unusual mushroom: it germinates inside a living organism, the larvae of certain kinds of moths, particularly the ghost moth or the bat moth (*Hepialus armoricanus*), which it mummifies, colonizes, and eventually kills.

The Latin etymology of *Cordyceps sinensis* is as follows: *cord* means "club," *ceps* means "head," and *sinensis* means "Chinese." The mushroom is also called the "caterpillar fungus" on account of its life cycle inside the larvae of the moth and is also called "winter worm, summer grass" because the ancient Chinese believed that the fungus was an animal in winter and a vegetable in summertime. Around 1850, Japanese herbalists began importing the mushroom from China and named it *tochukaso*, a Japanese translation of "winter worm, summer grass." The mushroom is sometimes called the "club-head fungus," a direct translation of its Latin name. The common name in China today is *dong chong xiaq cao* and in Tibet *yartsa gunbu*, both meaning "winter worm, summer grass," a poetic, if somewhat unusual, name for a medicinal mushroom.

There are over 680 documented varieties of *Cordyceps* mushroom, of which *Cordyceps sinensis* is but one. Many *Cordyceps* fungi grow by feeding on insect larvae and sometimes on mature insects. *Cordyceps* mushrooms grow on just about every category of insects: crickets, cockroaches, bees, centipedes, black beetles, and ants, to name just a few.

In appearance *Cordyceps sinensis* makes for an unusual sight. The mycelium is encased in the mummified body of the caterpillar, from which the fungus germinates. The fruit body, sprouting from the caterpillar, is shaped like a blade or twig, dark brown at the base and black at the top. Large fruit bodies sometimes branch out in the manner of antlers, so *Cordyceps* is sometimes called the "deer fungus." The mushroom is found in the wild at altitudes of 14,000 to 21,000 feet (4,500–7,000 meters). It grows in the alpine meadows of the Himalayas and other high mountain ranges of China, Tibet, Bhutan, and Nepal.

In 1996, mycologist Malcolm Clark accompanied members of the Mykot tribe as they foraged for *Cordyceps sinensis* in the Himalayas. The Mykots immigrated to Nepal long ago from Tibet. Like most Nepalese, they kept yaks, but the yaks are herded, not fenced. At a certain time of the year, when the snow melts, the yaks start heading up into the mountains and there is no way of holding them back. They climb up to 16,000 feet to find the *Cordyceps*. Clark was advised by his companions to eat *Cordyceps* to prevent altitude sickness and he ate fresh *Cordyceps* right out of the soil and was never sick.

As the tribesmen traveled with the yaks, they looked for a certain kind of primrose that blooms at high elevation. If the primrose is not blooming, the *Cordyceps* is not going to be out, and you may as well turn back because there will be no *Cordyceps* harvest. Fortunately, on that occasion, the primrose was in full bloom. The yaks ate the grass around the primrose flowers and the *Cordyceps*. The yaks also began mating.

Among mycologists, there is a debate as to whether the *Cordyceps* fungus grows outside the caterpillar or is ingested and grows from the inside. Clark believes that the caterpillars actually ingested the *Cordyceps* spores. "When dissecting the caterpillars, I found color variation in the tissue always in more or less the same place," he writes. "That leads me to believe that the spore is ingested. You can actually see the spot of inoculation where germination takes place. I can always find one spot on the larvae, which is softer and a different color, so what I'm proposing is that it is ingested and it germinates from the inside, where it grows like a tuber. It splits the caterpillar's head and grows out from there. When the ground starts to warm in the spring, the *Cordyceps* breaks through the ground and the mushroom appears."

The Mykots make a yogurt out of *Cordyceps*. They milk the yaks, skim the fat from the milk, and soak dried *Cordyceps* in the milk overnight. In the morning, the milk turns to yogurt. "Some of the collection spots we went to are hundreds of years old," Clark said about his expedition. "I accompanied the Mykots on the condition that I would not reveal where they harvest the *Cordyceps*. These were secret areas and I'm sure they would have liked to blindfold me on one or two occasions. It was a wonderful experience to be part of this ancient ritual."

For many centuries, *Cordyceps sinensis* occupied an important place as a tonic herb in the pharmacopoeia of traditional Chinese medicine. The West's first encounter with *Cordyceps* occurred in the early eighteenth century when Father Jean Baptiste Perennin du Halde, a Jesuit priest, brought specimens from China back to his native France. During his stay at the court of the Chinese emperor, Father Perennin took a lively interest in *Cordyceps*. Very likely, his curiosity about the mushroom came about when he himself was prescribed it during a grave illness. According to his diary, Father Perennin was very ill but had the good fortune to come upon an emissary to the Great Palace, who happened to be delivering *Cordyceps*. The emissary offered some of the herb to Father Perennin and he soon recovered.

In his diary, Father Perennin wrote that *Cordyceps* can "strengthen and renovate the powers of the system that have been reduced by overexertion or long sickness." He noted how rare *Cordyceps*

was in China, how it had to be imported from the mountain kingdom of Tibet, and how it was worth four times its weight in silver.
Upon his return to France, Father Perennin published an account
of his experiences with *Cordyceps* and the beneficial effects it had
on his own health. The report caused a small sensation within the
French scientific community, not least because it was the first
report of a fungus parasitizing an insect.

In 1843, the Reverend Dr. M.I. Berkeley, writing in the *New York
State Journal of Medicine,* reported in detail about the mysterious
"insect-plant." Dr. Berkeley noted that the root of *Cordyceps* is
indeed a caterpillar, but that the caterpillar had been taken over
almost entirely by the mushroom's mycelium. *Cordyceps* probably
made its debut in the United States in the middle of the nineteenth
century when Chinese immigrants began arriving to build the rail-
roads and brought their herbal medicines with them. Records
showed that Chinese physicians were prescribing *Cordyceps* in Ore-
gon and Idaho.

Into the twenty-first century, *Cordyceps* continues to be a highly prized herbal medicine in China, with extensive research conducted on the active ingredients, the differences among the
varieties, and the best methods of cultivation and extraction. Wild
Cordyceps is also highly valued. It is used especially to treat respiratory diseases, including lung cancer, where it is known to ameliorate a variety of symptoms of advanced disease.

In June 2006, John Holliday, director of research for Aloha Med-
icinals, a medicinal mushroom company based in Hawaii and California, led one of the first formal, Western scientific research
expeditions into the high country of Tibet in search of new strains
of *Cordyceps.* His group discovered what appear to be five previously unknown species, either closely related to *Cordyceps sinensis*
or only subspecies or strains of this fungus. Or they may appear
different because they are growing on other species of caterpillars.
The remote villagers and nomads in the region knew of these different types, and even had different names for them. Each type is
ranked in terms of medicinal usage and value. *Cordyceps* that grow
on white caterpillars is known as *Bu Carpo* in Tibetan and is the
lowest grade. *Cordyceps* that grows on a red-eyed caterpillar, called
Go Marpu, is considered better than *Bu Carpo* but not as good as the

top-quality grade, which is known locally as *Yartsa Gunbu*. There are also two other lower grades that are more uncommon and do not have their own Tibetan names. Dr. Holliday has managed to cultivate all of these types in the laboratory and is currently investigating their various chemical and biological properties.

Dr. Holliday is also conducting research into *Cordyceps* from other areas of the world, particularly the high Andes Mountains in Peru. There are about 250 newly found species of *Cordyceps* from Peru that have yet to be named by science. Some of these Peruvian *Cordyceps* have shown potent antibacterial and antiviral activities and are the subject of current research for the development of a new generation of nontoxic drugs for treating HIV/AIDS. Just how these species of *Cordyceps*, far remote from the classic Tibetan varieties, relate to one another is one of the questions being looked into.

11

The Quest for Common Ground

A t the beginning of the twenty-first century, we look back on more than a quarter century of China's opening up to the world. During this time, China has changed dramatically and irrevocably from an economically backward, closed society to become one of the great players on the international stage. China's economy now ranks third or fourth in the world and during the past year China's total expenditure on research and development is the world's second largest, behind only that of the United States. China has just announced the establishment of a state investment agency with $1 trillion of its foreign currency reserves, which is growing by $20 billion every month. Some of that money will be invested in research in biotechnology and medicine. The country has embraced Western science and Western medicine. In some Chinese cities, such as Beijing and Wuhan, there are one million university graduates each year. But to what extent will the West embrace the Chinese contribution to world culture and world medicine?

RESISTANCE TO CHANGE

There are many reasons to be optimistic. Like it or not, we live in an age of globalization. Today, there are very few who are not exposed to other cultures, and cultural curiosity is a hallmark of our age. But within the mainstream medical community, there is still resistance to the emergence of traditional Chinese medicine as an "alternative," even for (or particularly for) patients for whom Western medicine has failed. We believe that this impulse of resistance can, and must, change.

What are the components of this resistance? In the first place, some practices, such as acupuncture, Qigong, and Tai chi, may be seen as possessing a peculiarly Chinese cultural strangeness. Indeed, the Chinese are very proud of their traditional medicine and see it as an integral part of their cultural heritage. But what is cultural heritage and who owns it? In 1970, a UNESCO (United Nations Educational, Scientific, and Cultural Organization) conference stipulated that "cultural property constitutes one of the basic elements of civilization and . . . it is essential for every state to become alive to the moral implications to respect its own cultural heritage." But unlike a Greek vase or a Nigerian sculpture, traditional Chinese medicine as a cultural heritage is a movable feast—it does not have to stay in one place.

In "How China Became Chinese," a chapter in *Guns, Germs, and Steel,* evolutionary biologist Jared Diamond argued that China had favorable climate and geographical features as well as plant and animal species suitable for domestication. These factors taken together, rather than any particular genius of the Chinese people, made civilization possible. Perhaps any other ethnic group, given the same favorable conditions, would have done as well. This is not to say that Chinese culture does not "belong" to the Chinese, who are the custodians of that culture. Rather, what we are saying is that *all* culture also belongs to the whole human race.

In today's "global village," culture, although retaining its ethnic (but not ethnocentric) context, is increasingly seen as universal. The Nigerian philosopher Kwame Appiah puts it well in *Whose Culture Is It?*: "My people—human beings—made the Great Wall of China, the Sistine Chapel, the Chrysler Building: these things were made by creatures like me, through the exercise of skills and imagination." Chinese medicine as culture is like Chinese cuisine: something that can be shared. Indeed, in China the two often merge into each other, as there are many restaurants where delicious food is cooked with medicinal herbs.

A second problem is more troublesome. The system of Chinese medicine is founded without the underpinnings of Western science, suggesting that an alternative system of explanation of natural phenomena might also have validity. Thus, although some Chinese therapeutic interventions (such as the use of arsenic trioxide to treat leukemia) could be brought inside the framework of scientific medicine and thus become part of Western medicine, it is possible that other modalities, such as pulse diagnosis and acupuncture, will continue to be outside science as understood by the inheritors of the European Enlightenment. For many people, however, it is just such "alternative" explanations that make alternative medicine attractive.

THEORY OF THE CORRECT VIEW

Most Chinese, being pragmatic, are blithely unaware of the quest for a unifying *theory of the correct view* of everything, which has been such an important feature of Western civilization. Throughout most of Chinese history, official philosophy comprised the three teachings of Confucianism, Taoism, and Buddhism. In fact, Marco Polo found not only these three teachings but also Islam and Nestorian Christianity tolerated in the thirteenth-century Chinese court. For China, the major historical example of the theory of the correct view of everything was Marxism, of which the Chinese mutant, Mao Zedong Thought, wrought havoc in the country through the Cultural Revolution. Toward the end of the Cultural Revolution, the reformer Deng Xiaoping famously said: "It doesn't matter whether the cat is black or white so long as it catches mice."

Perhaps Western philosophy has not always insisted on a unifying theory of the correct view—did not pluralism flourish in ancient Greece? In his insightful book *The Closing of the Western Mind,* Charles Freeman traced the end of philosophical and religious pluralism to Emperor Constantine's espousal of Christianity in the fourth century. An official church, enjoying state largesse, tax-free status, and the gift of land and monuments *must* be distinguished from alternative explanations of human experience, the universe, and everything—that is, an insistence on a single philosophical system of explanation. A modern unifying theory, based on science, was proposed by evolutionary biologist Edward

O. Wilson in his book *Consilence: The Unity of Knowledge:* that Enlightenment science in the guise of Darwinism should encompass not only the physical and biological sciences but also the social sciences and social policy. In Wilson's world, scientists would run society. Such fundamentalism (religious or scientific) would not, of course, tolerate alternative systems of healing such as Chinese medicine.

Many Western visitors to China are astonished at the admixture of contrasting, even contradictory ideas, none more astonishing than the combination of communism and capitalism into "socialism with Chinese characteristics." If these two can be combined, then integrating Western and Chinese medicine is no big deal. For the Chinese, the Western quest for a theory of the correct view of everything is frankly odd and somewhat illogical. If a theory can explain some things, fine. If it can explain many things, it is even better. But how can a theory make claims on phenomena that it has not, or at least not yet, explained? How can a black cat explain a white cat?

This question is at the heart of the matter in the debate about alternative medicine. To many (though not all) practitioners, alternative medicine is about alternative theories as well as practice. In China, "integrative medicine" means integrating the practice of Western and Chinese medicine, while alternative theories are allowed space to flourish or perish according to their merits. It is, above all, *not* a world of "for us or against us."

It is well to point out that conventional medicine has its critics in the West, where its underpinnings are not entirely accepted within academic philosophy. This is particularly true of its approach to mental illness, which has been eloquently critiqued by philosopher Michel Foucault in *Madness and Civilization* and *The Birth of the Clinic,* by Thomas Szasz in *Ideology and Insanity,* and by R.D. Laing in *The Politics of Experience.* In his book *The Limits of Medicine,* Ivan Illich (1926–2002) described the medical transformation of death, a part of universal human experience, into "terminal ceremonies . . . therapy reaches its apogee in the death dance around the terminal patient . . . beds are filled with bodies neither dead nor alive." This is a scenario familiar to oncologists and their cancer patients. It is against this background that alternative methods of healing find their rapport with suffering humanity. The bitter truth is that Western medicine does not work very well against most forms of advanced cancer. Where it does work, as in leukemia, lymphoma, and some forms of childhood cancer, there is no debate but that it should be the modality of choice. This is also true in China. The problem concerns only the mice that the black cat cannot catch.

FINDING COMMON GROUND

Fortunately, things are changing. It is becoming increasingly recognized that there is no ineluctable conflict between mainstream Western medicine and alternative traditions of healing, except in the minds of a small minority of fundamentalists. This does not mean that there is no debate whatsoever between the East and West on the art of healing, but the debate in future will take place on a far more sophisticated level than it has in the past. The diverse traditions will have space to inform one another.

The Italian health minister, Livia Turco, recently said that she would do more to promote traditional Chinese medicine in her country and in the European Union (EU), and that Italy would issue licenses to practitioners of traditional Chinese medicine in the near future. In 2003, the U.S. Food and Drug Administration agreed that herbal medicines that have long been used could be registered as drugs even without clear chemical compositions, as long as they can be backed by good clinical data and quality stability. In 2004, the EU passed a law stipulating that, by 2011, herbal medicines sold in Europe can be registered as drugs. In 2006, China announced its intention to bid for a United Nations listing of its traditional medicine as a World Intangible Cultural Heritage.

We have found much common ground between traditional Chinese medicine and Western medicine. This is true even for the most "cutting-edge" Western medicine. The boundary between Western and Chinese medicine is getting blurred. There are about 100,000 Chinese scientists working in the West and those working in China are increasingly working in an area that can only be described as common ground. A very good example is the discovery by Professor Wang Zhen-yi and his group in Shanghai of the treatment for acute promyelocytic leukemia using differentiating agents. Instead of killing the leukemic cells, these drugs cause them to differentiate and become more like normal cells. This successful strategy has now been fully incorporated into Western medicine. One major impulse behind this strategy was that the ingredients were inexpensive, based on compounds related to vitamin A and arsenic trioxide. Although China's economy is growing rapidly, many people, especially in the rural areas, still have low incomes, so an affordable treatment is a high priority. This is also true for much of the rest of the world.

Another major area of common ground is immune therapy for cancer, based on a consideration of the host environment. It is very striking how the most advanced research in the West is now also focused on harnessing the body's immune response to fight cancer, something that is close to the basic idea of the Chinese approach to cancer. Of course, modern Western science has vastly more powerful tools to study the immune system and biotechnology has the means to apply this new knowledge, so that we can be confident that in the not too distant future, scientific immunotherapy can succeed where cruder treatment methods have failed. We only hope that when such breakthroughs occur, they can benefit the vast majority of cancer sufferers instead of just the few who can afford the treatment. This new cancer medicine must not be like a trip into space, a technologically feasible but economically nonviable dream.

For now, integrative oncology works very well in China, but it is done the other way around—an initially small but increasingly important body of Western medical knowledge and practice is integrated into an existing tradition of empirical observation and, to Western observers, alternative explanations of the body's functions.

A THERAPY OF HOPE

In this book, we have given prominent focus to the use of mushrooms in the treatment of cancer, which is prevalent not only in China, but also in Korea and Japan. This mushroom-based herbal medicine has a foundation of over a thousand years of empirical observations, but it was only recently that the domestication of mushrooms and the large-scale manufacture of their products became possible. Domestication of wild species is, in fact, a very complex process and has played an important part in the history of the human race. Of the millions of species of animals and plants in nature, only a small number have the right genetic makeup to become closely associated, in a mutually beneficial way, with human beings. We only have to think of the domestication of the horse and cattle, of wheat and rice, to know how profound the effects of domestication can be. Of course, it is too early to say that the domestication of mushrooms will have an equally beneficial effect, but it is indeed possible. What we know of the medicinal properties of mushrooms may be just the tip of the iceberg for future medical therapies. These advances are exciting, and people interested in the problem of cancer should work together, East and West. Some cultural and philosophical barriers, rather than objections based on medical sciences, may need to be overcome, but the core knowledge now being diffused offers a therapy of hope for the future.

Glossary

Acute. The term used classically to described cases of leukemia of short duration or rapid onset. In the modern context, the term remains useful although many cases of "acute" leukemia are now of longer duration, and even cured.

Acute lymphoblastic leukemia (ALL). The most common form of acute leukemia in children, less frequently affecting adults. The malignant cell in ALL is an immature cell of the lymphoid system.

Acute myeloid leukemia (AML). The most common form of acute leukemia in adults, less frequently affecting children. The malignant cell in AML is an immature cell of the bone marrow.

Antibody. A soluble protein molecule produced and secreted by B cells of the immune system in response to an antigen; it is capable of binding to that specific antigen.

Antibody-dependent cell-mediated cytotoxicity (ADCC). An immune response in which antibodies, by coating target cells, make the target cells vulnerable to attack by immune cells.

Antigen. Any substance that, when introduced into the body, is recognized by the immune system. Antigens have to be exposed to the immune system by specialized antigen-presenting cells, such as dendritic cells. The result of immune recognition is the priming of T lymphocytes or the production of antibody by B lymphocytes.

Apheresis. The separation of cells, usually by automated continuous flow systems. In such systems, blood flows from a vein into an

apheresis instrument that retains the cells of choice, such as lymphocytes or stem cells, and returns the rest of the blood cells and plasma
to the patient or donor.

Agaricus blazei, Agaricus subrufescens (Agaricus blazei). A mushroom species, sometimes known as *himematsutake* or a number of
other names. *Agaricus blazei* is edible, with a damp, sweet taste that
reminds some people of the flavor of almonds. Originally from a
small mountain town in Brazil called Piedade, located 120 miles
southeast of São Paulo, it also grows in the southeastern United
States. Many scientists believe that the active ingredients in *Agaricus
blazei* are more potent than that of any other mushrooms. It has shown
promise as an immunomodulator and a defense against tumors.

Autoimmune disease. A condition in which the body's immune system attacks its own tissues by directing antibodies or cells targeted
at the tissue's cells. These antibodies are termed auto-antibodies.
Common autoimmune diseases include rheumatoid arthritis, lupus,
and type 1 diabetes.

B cells. Small white blood cells crucial to the immune defenses. Also
known as B lymphocytes, they are derived from bone marrow and
develop into plasma cells that are the source of antibodies.

Beta cells. Cells in the pancreas that produce insulin. Transplantation
of cultured beta cells is a potential cell therapy for type 1 diabetes.

Beta-glucans. Beta-glucan molecules (-glucans) are one configura-
tion of polysaccharides, molecules known to stimulate the immune
response. Beta-glucans are found in abundance in mushrooms and
are one reason why they strengthen the immune system. The term
beta-glucan refers to the way that the sugar units are attached to one
another in the polysaccharide chain. Each glucose molecule has six
carbons, and the linkage between the different carbons can occur at
any position. A polysaccharide in which the molecule at the first
position is linked to the next molecule at the third position is called
a 1-3 beta-glucan. Most beta-glucans in mushrooms are of the 1-3
variety; plants, by contrast, mostly contain 1-4 beta-glucans.

Biotechnology. The use of living organisms or their products to make
or modify a substance. Biotechnology includes recombinant DNA
techniques (genetic engineering) and hybridoma technology.

Bone marrow. Soft tissue located in the cavities of the bones, particularly the skull, the sternum, and the long bones. The bone marrow is a vital organ of the blood-forming (hematopoietic) and immune systems and is the source of all blood cells.

Cell membrane. The outer "skin" of a cell. It is biologically very active and contains numerous receptors, which have the function of switching on or off many of the cell's functions. These receptor switches also communicate with one another and fine-tune or amplify their messages. They also communicate with receptors and other switch mechanisms within the cell.

Cellular immunity. Immune protection provided by the direct action of immune cells (as distinct from soluble molecules such as antibodies). Frequently, groups of cells such as dendritic cells, memory T cells, cytotoxic T cells, and natural killer cells are involved in a complex interplay of immune defense.

Chromosomes. Physical structures in the cell's nucleus that are composed of long strings of genes. Each human cell has 23 pairs of chromosomes, including one pair of sex chromosomes. A male has an X and a Y chromosome whereas a female has two X chromosomes. The other 22 pairs are called autosomes.

Chronic lymphocytic leukemia (CLL). The most common type of leukemia, mainly affecting older people. It generally runs a slow course over many years. The malignant cell in CLL is a mature-looking small lymphocyte.

Chronic myeloid leukemia (CML). Leukemia characterized by an initial insidious or chronic phase, usually followed by an abrupt transition to an aggressive form. CML is caused by a specific abnormality in the DNA of the cell in which two genes are translocated (juxtaposed) together, the bcr-ABL translocation. This usually results in an abnormal chromosome called the Philadelphia chromosome, although sometimes the changes can be more subtle and are discovered only by molecular techniques.

Clone. A group of genetically identical cells or organisms descended from a single common ancestor. The term is also used to describe the biotechnology process to reproduce multiple identical copies of genes, proteins, or cells.

Complement. A system of proteins that interact in a cascade manner, which helps to modulate and enhance the innate immune response.

Cord blood. Blood collected from the umbilical cord and placenta following delivery. Cord blood is a valuable source of stem cells. Cord blood banks store many thousands of units of cord blood and make them available for transplantation. In some cases, cord blood stem cells can be used instead of bone marrow stem cells for transplantation in the treatment of cancer and genetic disorders.

Cordyceps. In Latin, *cord* means "club," *ceps* means "head," and *sinensis* means "Chinese." The mushroom is also called the "caterpillar fungus" on account of its origin and, less frequently, "winter worm, summer plant." The mycelium is encased in the mummified body of the caterpillar, from which the fungus germinates. The fruit-body is capless, shaped like a blade or twig, dark brown at the base, and black at the top. *Cordyceps* grows in the alpine meadows of the Himalayas and other high mountain ranges of China, Tibet, and Nepal.

Co-stimulation. The delivery of a second signal from an antigen-presenting cell, such as a dendritic cell, to a T cell. The second signal rescues the activated T cell from a state of non-reactivity, allowing it to produce additional T cells. It is now known that co-stimulation is itself a complex interplay of cellular signals that modulates or fine-tunes the immune response.

Cytokines. Soluble molecules that the body produces to regulate responses between cells; for example, in reaction to viral and bacterial infections. These molecules assist in the orderly operation of the body's defense responses and include such proteins as interferons and interleukins.

Cytotoxic. Cell-killing ability; usually applied to drugs that kill cells capable of undergoing division, but also sometimes applied to cells themselves.

Cytotoxic T cells. A subset of T lymphocytes that can kill body cells infected by viruses or transformed by cancer.

Dendritic cells. White blood cells found in the spleen and other lymphoid organs. Dendritic cells typically use threadlike tentacles to enmesh antigens, which they present to T cells.

Diabetes. A disease in which there is failure of insulin production or function, including insulin resistance. Type 1 diabetes typically affects children and young adults and is a disease potentially treatable by cell therapy.

DNA (Deoxyribonucleic acid). A nucleic acid that is found in the cell nucleus. DNA is the carrier of genetic information.

Embryo. In the context of this book, the earliest life form following conception.

Embryonic stem cells. Cells obtained from the inner cell mass of the embryo, usually 4-6 days after conception. Embryonic stem cells can be cultured indefinitely in the laboratory and have the properties of self-renewal and differentiation into cells of many lineages.

Enzyme. A protein produced by living cells that promotes the chemical processes of life without itself being altered.

Fetus. A later stage of development of the product of conception compared with the embryo, when organs and tissues have begun to form.

Ganoderma lucidum (reishi* or *lingzhi). Reishi has been called the king of herbal medicines, with many herbalists ranking it above ginseng. The mushroom is usually taken for medicinal purposes only, as it has a very bitter, woody taste. *Ganoderma lucidum* is from the Latin words *gan*, which means "shiny," *derm* meaning "skin," and *lucidum* meaning "brilliant." Also called the "ten-thousand-year mushroom" and the "mushroom of immortality." It has a shiny, lacquered look and a kidney-shaped cap; sometimes the spores appear on the cap and give the appearance of sandpaper. It is found in dense, humid coastal provinces of China, and favors the decaying stumps of chestnut, oak, and other broad-leaf trees.

Gene. A unit of genetic material (DNA) that carries the directions a cell uses to perform a specific function, such as making a given protein.

Ginkgo biloba. Ginkgos are medium-large deciduous trees, reaching a height of 20-35 meters (66-115 feet), with an often angular crown and long, somewhat erratic branches. They are usually deep rooted and resistant to wind and snow damage. A combination of amazing disease resistance, insect-resistant wood, and the ability to form aerial roots and sprouts means that ginkgos are very long-lived, with some specimens claimed to be more than 2,500 years old. The extract of the ginkgo leaves contains flavonoid glycosides and terpenoids and has been used pharmaceutically. It is mainly used as memory enhancer and anti-vertigo agent.

Granulocyte colony-stimulating factor (G-CSF). A hemopoietic growth factor that has been found useful for stimulating stem cells for transplantation, with additional applications in cancer treatment.

Granulocyte-macrophage colony-stimulating factor (GM-CSF). A hemopoietic growth factor that has been found useful for stimulating immune responses, such as the growth of dendritic cells.

Grifola frondosa. Also known as hen of the woods, sheep's head, and maitake, it is an edible mushroom with a rippling form, no caps, and it grows in clusters at the foot of oak trees. The underground tubers from which hen of the woods arises has been used in traditional Chinese and Japanese medicine to enhance the immune system. Researchers have also indicated that whole maitake has the ability to regulate blood pressure, glucose and insulin, and lipids (cholesterol, triglycerides), and it may also be useful for weight loss.

Histocompatibility testing. A method of matching the self-antigens or human leukocyte antigens (HLAs) on the tissues of a transplant donor with those of the recipient. The closer the match, the better the chance that the transplant will succeed.

Human leukocyte antigens (HLA). Protein markers of "self" used in histocompatibility testing. Some HLA types also correlate with certain autoimmune diseases.

Hybridoma. A hybrid cell created by fusing an antigen-stimulated B lymphocyte with a long-lived neoplastic plasma cell. A hybridoma cell secretes a specific antibody called a monoclonal antibody.

Idiotype. The unique and characteristic parts of an antibody's variable region, which can themselves serve as antigens.

Immune response. The defensive reactions of the immune system.

Insulin. A hormone produced in the pancreas that is secreted into the bloodstream. It regulates blood sugar level and therefore plays an important role in metabolism.

Interferon. A family of biological agents that appears to be effective against some forms of leukemia, kidney cancer, and melanoma.

Interleukins. Messengers that are secreted by one set of white blood cells to influence the action of other white blood cells. Interleukins are among the most powerful of cytokines.

Interleukin-2 (IL-2). A cytokine that has been found useful in treating kidney cancer and melanoma. It may have an important role in blood and bone marrow transplantation and in immune therapy in general.

Leukemia. A classical term coined in the nineteenth century to describe a rapidly fatal disease characterized by the white appearance of part of the blood when allowed to stand, hence its literal meaning "white blood." Although we now know the many genetic abnormalities of leukemic cells that result in the many types of blood cancer, the appellations acute lymphoblastic leukemia (ALL), acute myeloid leukemia (AML), chronic lymphocytic leukemia (CLL), and chronic myeloid leukemia (CML) have been retained.

Leukocytes. White blood cells.

Lingzhi. See *Ganoderma lucidum*

Lymph. A slightly milky, yellowish fluid that carries lymphocytes, bathes the body tissues, and drains into the lymphatic vessels.

Lymphocytes. Small white blood cells produced in the lymphoid organs and paramount in the immune defenses.

Lymphoid organs. Organs of the immune system. They include the bone marrow, thymus, lymph nodes, spleen, and various other clusters of lymphoid tissue. The blood vessels and lymphatic vessels can also be considered lymphoid organs.

Lymphokine-activated killer (LAK) cells. Lymphocytes transformed in the laboratory by culture with cytokines, such as IL-2. LAK cells can attack tumor cells.

Maitake. See *Grifola frondosa*

Macrophages. Important cells of the immune system found in blood and tissues. They are capable of ingesting other cells or bacteria as well as functioning as antigen-presenting cells.

Major histocompatibility complex (MHC). A group of genes important in the control of several aspects of the immune response. MHC genes are expressed on all body cells and code for markers for the recognition of "self."

Metastasis. The passage of malignant cells around the body from their site of origin to establish new cancers elsewhere. Metastasis is now known to be not a simple passive process but a complex interplay of cellular receptors and other molecules with their counterparts in the target tissue microenvironment. Formation of new blood vessels is a critical part of this process in which changes on the genetic level of the cells play an important role.

Molecule. The smallest amount of a specific chemical substance that can exist alone. To break a molecule down into its constituent atoms is to change its character; a molecule of water, for instance, reverts to oxygen and hydrogen.

Monoclonal antibodies. Antibodies produced by a single cell (or its identical progeny) that are specific for a given antigen. As a tool for binding to specific protein molecules, monoclonal antibodies are invaluable in research, medicine, and industry.

Monocytes. White blood cells that are capable of differentiating into macrophages.

Mycelium. The vegetative part of a fungus consisting of a mass of branching, threadlike hyphae below the ground or within another substrate. It is through the mycelium that a fungus absorbs nutrients from its environment. Mycelium is also a vital component in many ecosystems: it helps increase the efficiency of water and nutrient absorption by many plants and it also is vital to the decomposition of plant material to form the organic part of soil and to release carbon dioxide back into the atmosphere.

Natural killer (NK) cells. Large granule-filled lymphocytes that destroy tumor cells and infected body cells. They are known as "natural" killers because they attack without first having to recognize specific antigens.

Nucleic acids. Large, naturally occurring molecules composed of chemical building blocks known as nucleotides. There are two kinds of nucleic acid, deoxyribonucleic acid (DNA) and ribonucleic acid (RNA).

Oncogene. Activated form of a proto-oncogene that is directly involved in causing malignant growth.

Organism. An individual living thing.

Peptidoglycan. Also known as murein, it is a polymer consisting of sugars and amino acids that forms a homogeneous layer outside the plasma membrane of eubacteria. Some Archaea have a similar layer of pseudopeptidoglycan.

Philadelphia chromosome. An abnormal chromosome in the leukemia cells of most patients with chronic myeloid leukemia (CML) and also a minority of patients with acute lymphoblastic leukemia (ALL).

Platelets. Granule-containing cellular fragments critical for blood clotting and sealing of wounds. They also contribute to the immune response.

Polysaccharides. Sometimes called glycans, these are relatively complex carbohydrates made up of many monosaccharides joined together by glycosidic linkages. They are therefore very large, often branched, molecules. They tend to be amorphous, insoluble in water, and have no sweet taste.

Proteins. Organic compounds made up of amino acids, they are one of the major constituents of plant and animal cells.

Proto-oncogene. Genes that have the ability to lead to a disturbed growth pattern, which can, in turn, lead to a malignant growth. Proto-oncogenes are made up of sequences of DNA that are susceptible to mutation.

Sanctuary sites. Areas of the body that are difficult for anti-leukemia drugs to reach.

Shiitake (*Lentinula edodes*). An edible mushroom native to East Asia. Shiitake mushrooms have been researched for their medicinal benefits, most notably their anti-tumor properties in laboratory mice. These studies, the earliest dating back to 1969, have also identified the polysaccharide lentinan, a 1-3 beta-glucan, as the active compound.

Spinal fluid. The fluid surrounding the brain and spinal cord.

Spores. A reproductive structure that is adapted for dispersion and surviving for extended periods of time in unfavorable conditions.

Spores form part of the life cycles of many plants, algae, fungi, and some protozoans.

Stem cells. Cells with unlimited renewal potential; these include hematopoietic stem cells, from which all blood cells derive. The bone marrow is rich in hematopoietic stem cells. Non-hematopoietic stem cells from bone marrow or blood may be utilized for repair of heart and other tissues.

T cells. Small white blood cells that orchestrate and/or directly participate in the immune defenses. Also known as T lymphocytes, they are processed in the thymus gland and secrete messenger molecules called lymphokines.

Thymus. A primary lymphoid organ, located high in the chest, where T lymphocytes proliferate and mature.

Tissue typing. See *Histocompatibility testing*

Tolerance. A state of non-responsiveness to a particular antigen or group of antigens.

Trametes versicolor. Formerly known as *Coriolus versicolor*, this is a common polypore mushroom of the genus *Trametes. Versicolor* means "of several colors" and this mushroom is found in a wide variety of colours. Some of its components—PSK or PSP—are used in cancer patients.

Tumor. Literally a swelling, but commonly used to mean a mass of cancer cells.

Tumor-infiltrating lymphocytes (TILs). These immune cells are extracted from the tumor tissue, treated in the laboratory, and re-infused into a patient with cancer.

Virus. A submicroscopic particle that can cause infectious disease. They can only reproduce in living cells.

Yunzhi. See *Trametes versicolor*

References

Introduction

American Cancer Society. *American Cancer Society's Guide to Complementary and Alternative Cancer Methods.* Atlanta, GA: American Cancer Society, 2000.

Boon, H., S. Westlake, R. Gray, et al. "Use of Complementary/Alternative Medicine by Men Diagnosed with Prostate Cancer: Prevalence and Characteristics." *Urology* 62 (2003): 849–853.

Cassileth, B., and G. Deng. "Complementary and Alternative Therapies for Cancer." *Oncologist* 9 (2004): 80–89.

DiGianni, L., J. Garber, E. Winer. "Complementary and Alternative Medicine Use Among Women with Breast Cancer." *J Clin Oncol* 20 (2002): 34–38.

Eisenberg, D., R. Davis, S. Ettner. "Trends in Alternative Medicine Use in the United States." *JAMA* 280 (1998): 1569–1575.

Ernst, E., and B. Cassileth. "The Prevalence of Complementary/Alternative Medicine in Cancer: A Systematic Review." *Cancer* 83 (1998): 777–782.

Gabor, Miklos, G.G., and P.J. Baird. "Curing Cancer: Running on Vapor." *GEN* (May 1, 2007): 6-10.

Kuhn, T. *Structure of Scientific Revolutions.* Chicago: University of Chicago Press, 1962.

M.D. Anderson Cancer Center. www.mdanderson.org.

Memorial Sloan-Kettering Cancer Center. www.mskcc.org.

National Cancer Institute, Office of Cancer Complementary and Alternative Medicine (NCI:OCCAM). www.cancer.gov/occam/.

133

National Center for Complementary and Alternative Medicine. www.nccam.nih.gov.

Natural Medicine Comprehensive Database. www.naturaldatabase.com.

Richardson, M., T. Sanders, J. Palmer, et al. "Complementary/Alternative Medicine Use in a Comprehensive Cancer Center and the Implications on Oncology." *J Clin Oncol* 18 (2000): 2505–2514.

Rosenthal, D.S., and E. Dean-Clower. "Integrative Medicine in Hematology/Oncology: Benefits, Ethical Considerations, and Controversies." *Hematology* (2005): 491–497.

Chapter 1: Times of Hope

Abeloff, M. (ed.). *Clinical Oncology,* 2nd ed. New York: Churchill Livingstone, 2000.

Balmain, A. "Cancer Genetics: From Boveri and Mandel to Microarrays." *Nature Rev Cancer* 1:1 (2001): 77–82.

Chabner, B.A., and T.G. Roberts. "Timeline: Chemotherapy and the War on Cancer." *Nature Rev Cancer* 5:1 (2005): 65–72.

David, Ian, and John and Margaret Millar. *Cambridge Dictionary of Scientists,* 2nd ed. Cambridge: Cambridge University Press, 2002.

DeVita, V.T., S. Hellman, and S.A. Rosenberg. *Principles and Practice of Oncology,* 6th ed. Philadelphia: Lippincott, Williams and Wilkins, 2001.

Mughal, T., and J. Goldman. *Understanding Leukaemia and Related Cancers.* London: Blackwell Science, 1999.

Nathan, D., and F. Oski (eds.). *Hematology of Infancy and Childhood,* 6th ed. Philadelphia: WB Saunders, 2003.

Porter, R. (ed.). *Cambridge Illustrated History of Medicine.* Cambridge: Cambridge University Press, 1996.

Chapter 2: What is Disease?

Avedon, J.F., F. Meyer, N.D. Bolsokhoeva, et al. *Buddha's Art of Healing.* New York: Rizzoli, 1998.

Chaga Health Mushroom Webpage. www.healthmushroom.com.

Donden, Y. *Health Through Balance.* New York: Snow Lion, 1986.

Goleman, D. (ed.). *Healing Emotions.* Boston: Shambhala, 1997.

Halpern, G.M. *Healing Mushrooms.* Garden City Park, NY: Square One, 2007.

Halpern, G.M. *Cordyceps: China's Healing Mushroom.* New York: Avery, 1999.

Li, P. *Management of Cancer with Chinese Medicine*. New York: Donica, 2004.

Porter, R. (ed.). *Cambridge Illustrated History of Medicine*. Cambridge: Cambridge University Press, 1996.

PuraPharm. www.oncozac.com.

Roberts, J.M. *Penguin History of the World*. London: Penguin Books, 1992.

Selby, A. *Ancient and Healing Art of Chinese Herbalism*. London: Hamlyn, 1998.

Wang, Z. "Ham Wasserman Lecture: Treatment of Acute Leukemia by Inducing Differentiation and Apoptosis." *Hematology 2003* (2003).

Chapter 3: The Dark Valley

Carney, D.N. "Lung Cancer—Time to Move On From Chemotherapy." *New Engl J Med* 346 (2002): 126–128.

DeVita, V.T., S. Hellman, and S.A. Rosenberg. *Principles and Practice of Oncology*, 6th ed. Philadelphia: Lippincott, Williams and Wilkins, 2001.

Gabor, Miklos, G.G., and P.J. Baird. "Curing Cancer: Running on Vapor." *GEN* (May 1, 2007): 6-10.

Goulart, B.H., R.G. Martins, T.J. Lynch. "Twenty-two Years of Phase III Trials for Patients with Advanced Non–Small Cell Lung Cancer—Sobering Results." *J Clin Oncol* 19 (2001): 4089.

Hansen, H. (ed.). *Textbook of Lung Cancer*. London: Martin Dunitz, 2000.

Proctor, R.N. "Tobacco and the Global Lung Cancer Epidemic." *Nature Rev Cancer* 1:1 (2001): 82–86.

Sporn, N.B., and N. Suh. "Chemoprevention: An Essential Approach to Controlling Cancer." *Nature Rev Cancer* 2:7 (2002): 537–543.

Tweedale, G. "Asbestos and Its Lethal Legacy." *Nature Rev Cancer* 2:4 (2002): 311–315.

Waller, A., and N. Caroline (eds.). *Handbook of Palliative Care in Cancer*. Boston: Butterworth Heinemann, 2000.

Williams, D. "Cancer After Nuclear Fallout: Lessons from the Chernobyl Accident." *Nature Rev Cancer* 2:7 (2002): 543–549.

Chapter 4: A Visit to a Chinese Hospital

Adachi, Y., et al. "The Effect Enhancement of Cytokine Production by Macrophages Stimulated with 1,3 Beta-D-glucan, Grifolan, Isolated from *Grifola frondosa*." *Biol Pharm Bull* 17 (1994): 1554–1560.

Arora, D. *Mushrooms Demystified.* Berkeley, CA: Ten Speed Press, 1986.

Browder, I.W., et al. "Beneficial Effect of Enhanced Macrophage Function in Trauma Patients." *Ann Surg* 211 (1990): 605–613.

Cancer Research UK. "Medicinal Mushrooms and Cancer." Available online at: http://www.sci.cancerresearchuk.org/labs/med_mush/med_mush.html.

Clute, M. "Beta-glucan: The Little Branched-chain Polysaccharide that Might." *Natural Foods Merchandiser* 3 (2001): 21–24.

DiLuzio, N. "Immunopharmacology of Glucan: A Broad-spectrum Enhancer of Host Defense Mechanisms." *Trends Pharmacol* 4 (1983): 344–347.

Ellertsen, L.K., et al. "Effect of a Medicinal Extract from *Agaricus blazei Murill* on Gene Expression in Human Monocytes." Poster 1454 presented at the World Allergy Congress, München, Germany, June 26–30, 2005.

Fujimiya, Y., et al. "Selective Tumoricidal Effect of Soluble Proteoglucan Extracted from the Basidiomycete, *Agaricus blazei Murill,* Mediated via Natural Killer Cell Activation and Apoptosis." *Cancer Immunol Immunother* 46 (1998): 147–159.

Fujimiya, Y., et al. "Tumor-specific Cytocidal and Immunopotentiating Effects of Relatively Low Molecular Weight Products Derived from the Basidiomycete, *Agaricus blazei Murill.*" *Anticancer Res* 19 (1999): 113–118.

Fujimiya, Y., et al. "Peroral Effect on Tumour Progression of Soluble Beta-(1,6)-glucans Prepared by Acid Treatment from *Agaricus blazei. Murr.* (Agaricaceae, Higher Basidiomycetes)." *Int J Med Mushr* 2 (2000): 43–49.

Gibson, G., et al. "Dietary Modulation of the Human Colonic Microbiota: Introducing the Concept of Prebiotics." *J Nutr* 125 (1995): 1401–1412.

Halpern, G.M. *Healing Mushrooms.* Garden City Park, NY: Square One, 2007.

Hobbs, C. *Medicinal Mushrooms.* Santa Cruz, CA: Botanica Press, 1986.

Huddler, G. *Magical Mushrooms, Mischievous Molds.* Princeton, NJ: Princeton University Press, 1998.

Ito, H., et al. "Anti-tumor Effects of a New Polysaccharide-protein Complex (ATOM) Prepared from *Agaricus blazei* (Iwade Strain 101) and Its Mechanisms in Tumor-bearing Mice." *Anticancer Res* 17 (1997): 277–284.

Kim, Y.W., et al. "Anti-diabetic Activity of Beta-glucans and Their Enzymatically Hydrolyzed Oligosaccharides from *Agaricus blazei.*" *Biotechnol Lett* 27:7 (2005): 483–487.

Kimura, Y., et al. "Isolation of an Anti-angiogenic Substance from *Agaricus blazei Murrill:* Its Antitumor and Antimetastatic Actions." *Cancer Sci* 95:9 (2004): 758–764.

Lindequist, U., et al. "The Pharmacological Potential of Mushrooms." *eCAM* 2 (2005): 285–299.

Lui, E. "Free Radical Scavenging Activities of Mushroom Polysaccharide Extracts." *Life Sci* 60:10 (1997): 763–771.

Mansell, P.W., et al. "Macrophage-mediated Destruction of Human Malignant Cells *in vivo.*" *J Natl Cancer Inst* 54 (1975): 571–580.

Martensen, R. "Cancer: Medical History and the Framing of a Disease." *JAMA* 271 (1994): 24–28.

Mizuno, T., et al. "Antitumor Activity and Some Properties of Water-soluble Polysaccharides from "Himematsutake," the Fruiting Body of *Agaricus blazei Murrill.*" *Agr Biol Chem (Tokyo)* 54 (1990): 2889–2896.

Mizuno, T., et al. "Health Foods and Medicinal Usage of Mushrooms." *Food Rev Intern* 11 (1995): 69–81.

Mizuno, M., et al. "Polysaccharides from *Agaricus blazei* Stimulate Lymphocyte T-cell Subsets in Mice." *Biosci Biotechnol Biochem* 62 (1998): 434–437.

Mizuno, T., et al. "Anti-tumor Polysaccharide from the Mycelium of Liquid-cultured *Agaricus blazei Mill.*" *Biochem Mol Biol Int* 47:4 (1999): 707–714.

Nakagaki, T. "Intelligence: Maze-solving by an Amoeboid Organism." *Nature* 407 (2000): 123–125.

Ohno, N., et al. "Antitumor Beta-glucan from the Cultured Fruit-body of *Agaricus blazei.*" *Biol Pharm Bull* 24:7 (2001): 820–828.

Ohno, N., et al. "Effect of Beta-glucan on the Nitric Oxide Synthesis of Peritoneal Macrophage in Mice." *Biol Pharm Bull* 19 (1996): 608–612.

Ooi, V.E.C., et al. "A Review of Pharmacological Activities of Mushroom Polysaccharides." *Int J Med Mushr* 1 (1999): 195–206.

Reshetnikov, S.C., et al. "Higher Basidiomycetes as a Source of Antitumour and Immunostimulating Polysaccharides." *Int J Med Mushr* 3 (2001): 361–394.

Rodman, W.L. "Cancer: Its Etiology and Treatment." *Am Pract News* 16 (1893): 409–417.

Ross, G.D., et al. "Therapeutic Intervention with Complement and Betaglucan in Cancer." *Immunopharmacology* 42 (1999): 61–74.

Schaechter, E. *In the Company of Mushrooms.* Cambridge, MA: Harvard University Press, 1997.

Schaechter, E. "Weird and Wonderful Fungi." *Microbiol Today* 27 (2000): 116–117.

Sharon, N., et al. "Carbohydrates in Cell Recognition." *Scient Am J* (1993): 74–81.

Smith, M.L., et al. "The Fungus, *Armarillaria bulbosa,* is Among the Largest and Oldest Living Organisms." *Nature* 356 (1992): 428–431.

Stijve, T., et al. "*Agaricus blazei Murrill*—A New Gourmet and Medicinal Mushroom From Brazil." *Australasian Mycol* 21:1 (2002): 29–33.

Takaku, T., et al. "Isolation of an Antitumor Compound from *Agaricus blazei Murrill* and Its Mechanism of Action." *J Nutr* 131:5 (2001): 1409–1413.

Wasser, S.P. "Review of Medicinal Mushroom Advances: Good News from Old Allies." *HerbalGram* 56 (2002): 28–33.

Wasser, S.P., et al. "Medicinal Properties of Substances Occurring in Higher Basidiomycete Mushrooms: Current Perspectives." *Int J Med Mushr* 1 (1999): 31–62.

Wasser, S.P., et al. "Is a Widely Cultivated Culinary-medicinal Royal Sun *Agaricus* (The Himematsutake Mushroom) Indeed *Agaricus blazei Murrill?*" *Int J Med Mushr* 4 (2002): 267–290.

Wasson, R. Gordon. *Divine Mushroom of Immortality.* New York: Harcourt Brace Jovanovich, 1968.

Yue, D., et al. *Advanced Study for Traditional Chinese Herbal Medicine, Institute of Materia Medica.* Beijing, China: Medical University and China Peking Union Medical University Press, 1995.

Chapter 5: A Success Story

Ball, E.D., P. Law, and J.W. Lister: *Hematopoietic Stem Cell Therapy.* New York: Churchill Livingstone, 2000.

Hayhoe, Frank. *Leukaemia* (1960). This monograph is a source of material regarding early transplantation attempts and the recovery of the bone marrow from radiation injury.

Little, Marie-Terese, and Rainer Storb. "History of Hematopoietic Stem Cell Transplantation." *Nature Rev Cancer* 2:3 (2002): 231–238.

Reiffers, J., J.M. Goldman, and J.O. Armitage. *Blood Stem Cell Transplantation.* London: Martin Dunitz, 1998.

Chapter 6: Nature's Healing Gift

Adachi, Y., et al. "Enhancement of Cytokine Production by Macrophages Stimulated with 1-3 Beta-D-glucan, Grifolan (GRN), Isolated from *Grifola frondosa.*" *Biol Pharm Bull* 17 (1994): 1554–1560.

Bae, E.A., et al. "Effect of *Lentinus edodes* on the Growth of Intestinal Lactic Acid Bacteria." *Arch Pharmac Res* 20 (1997): 443–447.

Bratkovich, S.M. "Shiitake Mushroom Production: Obtaining Spawn, Obtaining and Preparing Logs, and Inoculation." Available online at: http://ohioline.osu.edu/for-fact/0040.html.

Cancer Research UK. "Medicinal Mushrooms and Cancer." Available online at: http://www.sci.cancerresearchuk.org/labs/med_mush/med_mush.html.

Chihara, G., et al. "Fractionation and Purification of the Polysaccharides with Marked Anti-tumor Activity, Especially Lentinan from *Lentinus edodes* (Berk.) Sing., an Edible Mushroom." *Cancer Res* 30 (1970): 2776–2781.

Fullerton, S.A., et al. "Induction of Apoptosis in Human Prostatic Cancer Cells with Beta-glucan (Maitake Mushroom Polysaccharide)." *Mol Urol* 4 (2000): 7–13.

Horio, H., et al. "Maitake (*Grifola frondosa*) Improves Glucose Tolerance of Experimental Diabetic Rats." *J Nutr Sci Vitaminol (Tokyo)* 47:1 (2001): 57–63.

Ikekawa, T., et al. "Anti-tumor Activity of Aqueous Extracts of Edible Mushrooms." *Cancer Res* 29 (1969): 734–735.

Jones, K. "Maitake: A Potent Medicinal Food." *J Altern Complement Ther* 4 (1998): 420–429.

Klurfeld, D.M. "Synergy Between Medical and Nutrient Therapies: George Washington meets Rodney Dangerfield." *J Am Coll Nutr* 20:5 Suppl (2001): 349S-353S.

Kodama, N., A. Asakawa, A. Inui, et al. "Enhancement of Cytotoxicity of NK Cells by D-fraction, a Polysaccharide from *Grifola frondosa*." *Oncol Rep* 13:3 (2005): 497–502.

Kodama, N., et al. "Can Maitake MD-fraction Aid Cancer Patients?" *Alt Med Rev* 7:3 (2002): 236–239.

Kubo, K., et al. "The Effect of Maitake Mushrooms on Liver and Serum Lipids." *Altern Ther Health Med* 2 (1996): 62–66.

Kurashige, S., et al. "Effects of *Lentinus edodes, Grifola frondosa* and *Pleurotus ostreatus* Administration on Cancer Outbreak, and Activities of Macrophages and Lymphocytes in Mice Treated with a Carcinogen, Nbutyl-N-butanolnitrosoamine." *Immunopharmacol Immunotoxicol* 19 (1997): 175–183.

Landis-Piwowar, K.R., et al. "Evaluation of Proteasome-inhibitory and Apoptosis-inducing Potencies of Novel (-)-EGCG Analogs and Their Prodrugs." *Int J Mol Med* 15:4 (2005): 735–742.

Lee, E.W., et al. "Suppression of D-galactosamine-induced Liver Injury by Mushrooms in Rats." *Biosci Biotechnol Biochem* 64 (2000): 2001–2004.

Mayell, M. "Maitake Extracts and Their Therapeutic Potential." *Altern Med Rev* 6:1 (2001): 48–60.

Minato, K., et al. "Influence of Storage Conditions on Immunomodulating Activities of *Lentinus edodes.*" *Int J Med Mushr* 1 (1999): 243–250.

Mizuno, T. "Bioactive Biomolecules of Mushrooms: Food Functions and Medicinal Effects of Mushroom Fungi." *Food Rev Intern* 11 (1995): 7–21.

Mizuno, T., et al. "Maitake, *Grifola frondosa*: Pharmacological Effects." *Food Rev Int* 11 (1995): 135–149.

Nanba, H. "Maitake D-fraction: Healing and Preventive Potential for Cancer." *J Orthomol Med* 12 (1997): 43–49.

Nanba, H., et al. "Effects of Maitake (*Grifola frondosa*) Glucan in HIV-infected Patients." *Mycoscience* 41 (2000): 293–295.

Ng, M.L., et al.. "Inhibition of Human Colon Carcinoma Development by Lentinan from Shiitake Mushrooms (*Lentinula edodes*)." *J Altern Complement Med* 8:5 (2002): 581–589.

Nishida, I., et al. "Antitumour Activity Exhibited by Orally Administered Extracts from Fruit-body of *Grifola frondosa* (Maitake)." *Chem Pharmac Bull* 36 (1988): 1819–1827.

Ohno, N., et al. "Enhancement of LPS Triggered TNF-alpha (Tumor Necrosis Factor-alpha) Production by 1-3 Beta-D-glucan in Mice." *Biol Pharm Bull* 18 (1995): 126–133.

Ohtsuru, M. "Anti-obesity Activity Exhibited by Orally Administered Powder of Maitake Mushroom (*Grifola frondosa*)." *Anshin* 7 (1992): 198–200.

Okazaki, M., et al. "Structure-activity Relationship of 1-3 Beta-D-glucans in the Induction of Cytokine Production from Macrophages, *in vitro.*" *Biol Pharm Bull* 18 (1995): 1320–1327.

Stamets, P. *Mycelium Running: How Mushrooms Can Save the World.* Berkeley, CA: Ten Speed Press, 2005.

Suzuki, H., et al. "Inhibition of the Infectivity and Cytopathoc Effect of Human Immunodeficiency Virus by Water-soluble Lignin in an Extract of the Culture Medium of *Lentinus edodes* Mycelia (LEM)." *Biochem Biophys Res Comm* 160 (1989): 367–373

Yap, A.T., et al. "An Improved Method for the Isolation of Lentinan from the Edible and Medicinal Shiitake Mushroom, *Lentinus edodes* (Berk.) Sing. (Agaricomycetidae)." *Int J Med Mushr* 3 (2001): 6–19.

Yokota, M. "Observatory Trial of Anti-obesity Activity of Maitake (*Grifola frondosa*)." *Anshin* 7 (1992): 202–204.

Zhang, Y., et al. "Cyclooxygenase Inhibitory and Antioxidant Compounds from the Mycelia of the Edible Mushroom *Grifola frondosa*." *J Agric Food Chem* 50:26 (2002): 7581–7585.

Zhuang, C., et al. "Biological Responses from *Grifola frondosa* (Dick.:Fr.) S.F. Gray-Maitake (Aphyllophormycetideaea)." *Int J Med Mushr* 1 (1999): 317–324.

Chapter 7: New Beginnings

Carter, P. "Improving the Efficacy of Antibody-based Cancer Therapies." *Nature Rev Cancer* 1:2 (2001): 118–129.

"Molecular Targets in Cancer Therapy and Their Impact on Cancer Management." A report of the State of the Art Conference, Montreux, Switzerland, and published as a supplement to *Oncology* 63 (2002).

Rowe, J.M. *Hematology 2001* (2001).

Stern, P., P.L.C. Beverley, and M.W. Carroll (eds.). *Cancer Vaccines and Immunotherapy*. Cambridge: Cambridge University Press, 2000.

Chapter 8: *Lingzhi* and *Yunzhi*

El-Mekkawy, S., et al. "Anti-HIV-1 and Anti-HIV-1-protease Substances from *Ganoderma lucidum*." *Phytochemistry* 49 (1998): 1651–1657.

Fujimoto, S., et al. "Clinical Value of Immunochemotherapy with OK-432." *Jpn J Surg* 3 (1979): 190–196.

Fujita, R., J. Liu, K. Shimizu, et al. "Anti-androgenic Activities of *Ganoderma lucidum*." *J Ethnopharmacol* 102:1 (2005): 107–112.

Halpern, G.M. *Healing Mushrooms*. Garden City Park, NY: Square One, 2007.

Hayakawa, K., et al. "Effect of Krestin (PSK) as Adjuvant Treatment on the Prognosis after Radical Radiotherapy in Patients with Non–Small Cell Lung Cancer." *Anticancer Res* 13 (1993): 1815–1820.

Hong, S.G., et al. "Phylogenetic Analysis of *Ganoderma* Based on Nearly Complete Mitochondrial Small-subunit Ribosomal DNA Sequences." *Mycologia* 96 (2004): 742–755.

Hsu, H.Y., et al. "Extract of Reishi Polysaccharides Induces Cytokine Expression via TLR4-modulated Protein Kinase Signaling Pathways." *J Immunol* 173:10 (2004): 5989–5999.

Ikusawa, T., et al. "Fate and Distribution of an Anti-tumour Protein-bound Polysaccharide PSK (Krestin)." *Int J Immunopharmacol* 10 (1988): 415–423.

Iwatsuki, K., et al. "Lucidenic Acids P and Q, Methyl Lucidenate P, and Other Terpenoids from the Fungus *Ganoderma lucidum* and Their Inhibitory Effects on Epstein-Barr Virus Activation." *J Natural Prod* 66:12 (2003): 1582–1585.

Jian, Z.H., et al. "The Effect of PSP and LAK Cell Function." In Yang, Q.Y. (ed.). *Advanced Research in PSP.* Hong Kong: Hong Kong Association for Health Care, 1999, pp. 143–150.

Jiang, J., et al. "*Ganoderma lucidum* Suppresses Growth of Breast Cancer Cells Through the Inhibition of Akt/NF-kappa Signaling." *Nutr Cancer* 49:2 (2004): 209–216.

Jong, S., et al. "PSP—A Powerful Biological Response Modifier from the Mushroom *Coriolus versicolor.*" In Yang, Q.Y. (ed.). *Advanced Research in PSP.* Hong Kong: Hong Kong Association for Health Care, 1999, pp. 16–18.

Kaibarara, N., et al. "Postoperative Long-term Chemotherapy for Advanced Gastric Cancer." *Jpn J Surg* 6 (1976): 54–59.

Kidd, P.M. "The Use of Mushroom Glucans and Proteoglycans in Cancer Therapy." *Altern Med Rev* 5 (2000): 4–27.

Kim, K.C., et al. "*Ganoderma lucidum* Extracts Protect DNA from Strand Breakage Caused by Hydroxyl Radical and UV Irradiation." *Int J Mol Med* 4 (1999): 273–277.

Koch, J., et al. "The Influence of Selected Basidiomycetes on the Binding of Lipopolysaccharide to Its Receptor." *Int J Med Mushrooms* 4 (2002): 229–235.

Kondo, M., et al. "Evaluation of an Anticancer Activity of a Protein-bound Polysaccharide PSK (Krestin)." In Torisu, M., and T. Yoshida (eds.). *Basic Mechanisms and Clinical Treatment of Tumour Metastasis.* New York: Academic Press, 1985, pp. 623–636.

Lau, C.B., et al. "Cytotoxic Activities of *Coriolus versicolor* (*Yungzhi*) Extract on Human Leukemia and Lymphoma Cells by Induction of Apoptosis." *Life Sci* 75:7 (2004): 797–808.

Lin, S.B., et al. "Triterpene-enriched Extracts from *Ganoderma lucidum* Inhibit Growth of Hepatoma Cells via Suppressing Protein Kinase C, Activating Mitogen-activated Protein Kinases and G2-phase Cell Cycle Arrest." *Life Sci* 72:21 (2003): 2381–2390.

Lin, Z.B. "Focus on Anti-oxidative and Free Radical Scavenging Activity of *Ganoderma lucidum.*" *J Appl Pharmacol* 12 (2004): 133–137.

Lino, Y., et al. "Immunochemotherapies vs. Chemotherapy as Adjuvant Treatment after Curative Resection of Operable Breast Cancer." *Anticancer Res* 15 (1995): 2907–2912.

Liu, F., et al. "Induction in the Mouse of Gene Expression of Immunomodulating Cytokines by Mushroom Polysaccharide Complexes." *Life Sci* 58 (1996): 1795–1803.

Liu, J.X., et al. "Phase II Clinical Trial for PSP Capsules." *PSP International Symposium.* Shanghai, China: Fudan University Press, 1993.

Liu, J.X., et al. "Phase III Clinical Trial for *Yun Zhi* Polysaccharopeptide (PSP) Capsules." In Yang, Q.Y. (ed.). *Advanced Research in PSP.* Hong Kong: Hong Kong Association for Health Care, 1999, pp. 295–303.

Liu, L.F. "PSP in Clinical Cancer Therapy." In Yang, Q.Y. (ed.). *Advanced Research in PSP.* Hong Kong: Hong Kong Association for Health Care, 1999, pp. 68–75.

Lu, Q.Y., et al. "*Ganoderma lucidum* Extracts Inhibit Growth and Induce Actin Polymerization in Bladder Cancer Cells *in vitro.*" *Cancer Lett* 216:1 (2004): 9–20.

Lu, Q.Y., et al. "*Ganoderma lucidum* Spore Extract Inhibits Endothelial and Breast Cancer Cells *in vitro.*" *Oncol Rep* 12:3 (2004): 659–662.

Mao, X.W., et al. "Effects of Extract of *Coriolus versicolor* and IL-2 on Radiation Against Three Tumor Lines." Loma Linda University, unpublished data, 1998.

McCune, C.S., et al. "Basic Concepts of Tumour Immunology and Principles of Immunotherapy." In *Clinical Oncology,* 7th ed. Philadelphia: W.B. Saunders, 1993, p. 123.

Min, B.S., et al. "Triterpenes from the Spores of *Ganoderma lucidum* and Their Cytotoxicity Against Meth-A and LLC Tumor Cells." *Chem Pharm Bull (Tokyo)* 48:7 (2000): 1026–1033.

Min, B.S., et al. "Anticomplement Activity of Terpenoids from the Spores of *Ganoderma lucidum.*" *Planta Med* 67 (2001): 811–814.

Moncalvo, J.M., et al. "Phylogenetic Relationships in *Ganoderma* Inferred from the Internal Transcribed Spacers and 25S Ribosomal DNA Sequences." *Mycologia* 87 (1995): 223–238.

Morimoto, T., et al. "Postoperative Adjuvant Randomised Trial Comparing Chemoendocrine Therapy, Chemotherapy and Immunotherapy for Patients with Stage II Breast Cancer: 5-year Results from the Nishimihou Cooperative Study Group of Adjuvant Chemoendocrine Therapy for Breast Cancer (ACETBC) of Japan." *Eur J Cancer* 32A (1996): 235–242.

Nakazato, H., et al. "Efficacy of Immunochemotherapy as Adjuvant Treatment after Curative Resection of Gastric Cancer." *Lancet* 343 (1994): 1122–1126.

Ng, T.B., et al. "Polysaccharopeptide from the Mushroom *Coriolus versicolor* Possesses Analgesic Activity but Does Not Produce Adverse Effects on Female Reproduction or Embryonic Development in Mice." *Gen Pharmacol* 29 (1997): 269–273.

Ogoshi, K., et al. "Possible Predictive Markers of Immunotherapy in Oesophageal Cancer: Retrospective Analysis of a Randomised Study." *Cancer Invest* 13 (1995): 363–369.

Okazaki, M., et al. "Structure-activity Relationship of (1-3)-D-glucan in the Induction of Cytokine Production from Macrophages *in vitro.*" *Biol Pharmacol Bull* 18 (1995): 1320–1327.

Qian, Z.M., et al. "Polysaccharide Peptide (PSP) Restores Immunosuppression Induced by Cyclophosphamide." In Yang, Q.Y. (ed.). *Advanced Research in PSP.* Hong Kong: Hong Kong Association for Health Care, 1999, pp. 154–163.

Sakagami, H., et al. "Induction of Immunopotentiation Activity by a Protein-bound Polysaccharide, PSK." *Anticancer Res* 11 (1991): 993–1000.

Shiu, W.C.T., et al. "A Clinical Study of PSP on Peripheral Blood Counts During Chemotherapy." *Physiol Res* 6 (1992): 217–218.

Soo, T.S. "The Therapeutic Value of *Ganoderma lucidum.*" Abstract from the 8th International Mycological Congress, Vancouver, B.C., Canada, 1994.

Stanley, G., et al. "*Ganoderma lucidum* Suppresses Angiogenesis Through the Inhibition of Secretion of VEGF and TGF-beta1 from Prostate Cancer Cells." *Biochem Biophys Res Comm* 330:1 (2005): 46–52.

Stephens, L.C., et al. "Apoptosis in Irradiated Murine Tumours." *Radiation Res* 127 (1991): 308.

Sugimachi, K., et al. "Hormone Conditional Cancer Chemotherapy for Recurrent Breast Cancer Prolongs Survival." *Jpn J Surg* 14 (1994): 217–221.

Sun, Z., et al. "The Ameliorative Effect of PSP on the Toxic and Side Reaction of Chemo- and Radiotherapy of Cancers." In Yang, Q.Y. (ed.). *Advanced Research in PSP.* Hong Kong: Hong Kong Association for Health Care, 1999.

Toi, M., et al. "Randomised Adjuvant Trial to Evaluate the Addition of Tamoxifen and PSK to Chemotherapy in Patients with Primary Breast Cancer." *Cancer* 70 (1992): 2475–2483.

Tochikura, T.S., et al. "A Biological Response Modifier, PSK, Inhibits Human Immunodeficiency Virus Infection *in vitro.*" *Biochem Biophys Res Comm* 148 (1987): 726–733.

Tsang, K.W., et al. "*Coriolus versicolor* Polysaccharide Peptide Slows Progression of Advanced Non-small Cell Lung Cancer." *Resp Med* 97:6 (2003): 618–624.

Tsujitani, S., et al. "Postoperative Adjuvant Immunochemotherapy and Infiltration of Dendritic Cells for Patients with Advanced Gastric Cancer." *Anticancer Res* 12 (1992): 645–648.

Tsukagoshi, S., et al. "Krestin (PSK)." *Cancer Treat Rev* 11 (1984): 131–155.

Tzianabos, A. "Polysaccharide Immunomodulators as Therapeutic Agents: Structural Aspects and Biologic Functions." *Clin Microbiol Rev* 13 (2000): 523–533.

Wachtel-Galor, S., et al. "*Ganoderma lucidum* ("*Lingzhi*"), a Chinese Medicinal Mushroom: Biomarker Responses in a Controlled Human Supplementation Study." *Br J Nutr* 91:2 (2004): 171–173.

Wang, H., et al. "Ganodermin, an Antifungal Protein from Fruiting Bodies of the Medicinal Mushroom *Ganoderma lucidum.*" *Peptides* (July 20, 2005).

Wang, S.Y., et al. "The Anti-tumor *Ganoderma lucidum* is Mediated by Cytokines Released from Activated Macrophages and T Lymphocytes." *Int J Cancer* 70 (1997): 699–705.

Wasser, S.P. "Review of Medicinal Mushroom Advances: Good News from Old Allies." *HerbalGram* 56 (2002): 28–33.

Yang, Q.Y. (ed.). *Advanced Research in PSP.* Hong Kong: Hong Kong Association for Health Care, 1999.

Yao, W. "Prospective Randomised Trial of Radiotherapy Plus PSP in the Treatment of Oesophageal Carcinoma." In Yang, Q.Y. (ed.). *Advanced Research in PSP.* Hong Kong: Hong Kong Association for Health Care, 1999, pp. 310–313.

Yokoe, T., et al. "HLA Antigen as Predictive Index for the Outcome of Breast Cancer Patients with Adjuvant Immunochemotherapy with PSK." *Anticancer Res* 17 (1997): 2815–2818.

Yu, S., et al. "An Experimental Study on the Effects of *Lingzhi* Spore on the Immune Function and ^{60}Co Radioresistance in Mice." *J Natural Prod* 63:4 (2000): 514–516.

Zhong, B.Z., et al. "Genetic Toxicity Test of *Yun Zhi* Polysaccharide (PSP)." In Yang, Q.Y. (ed.). *Advanced Research in PSP.* Hong Kong: Hong Kong Association for Health Care, 1999, pp. 285–294.

Zhu, M., et al. "Triterpene Antioxidants from *Ganoderma lucidum.*" *Phytother Res* 13 (1999): 529–531.

Chapter 9: Invaders and Defenders

Bassett, Pamela. *Cell Therapy Technologies, Markets and Opportunities.* Further information is available online: www.drugsandmarket.com.

Chang, Alfred, et al. "Phase II Trial of Autologous Tumor Vaccination, Anti-CD3 Activated Vaccine Primed Lymphocytes and Interleukin-2 in Stage IV Renal Cell Cancer." *J Clin Oncol* 21:5 (2003).

Hoover Jr., H.C., J.S. Brandhorst, L.C. Peters, et al. "Adjuvant Active Specific Immunotherapy for Human Colorectal Cancer: 6.5-year Median Follow-up of a Phase II Prospectively Randomized Trial." *J Clin Oncol* 11 (1993): 390–399.

International Conference on Harmonization (ICH) publishes periodic Good Clinical Practice (GCP) guidelines on the conduct of clinical trials. These are available from the regulatory agencies of individual European countries, the U.S., and Japan.

Osband, M.E., P.T. Lavin, R.K. Babayan, et al. "Effect of Auto-lymphocyte Therapy on Survival and Quality of Life in Patients with Metastatic Renal Cell Carcinoma." *Lancet* 335 (1990): 994–998.

Pardoll, D., and J. Allison. "Cancer Immunotherapy—Breaking the Barriers to Harvest the Crop." *Nature Med* 10:9 (2004): 887–892.

Proceedings of the Fifth Annual Walker's Cay Colloquium on Cancer Vaccines and Immunotherapy. Albert Sabin Vaccine Institute (2003).

Proceedings of the 10th Annual Meeting of the International Society for Cellular Therapy. Available online at: www.celltherapy.org.

Rooney, C.M., C.A. Smith, C.Y. Ng, et al. "Infusion of Cytotoxic T Cells for the Prevention and Treatment of Epstein-Barr Virus–induced Lymphoma in Allogeneic Transplant Recipients." *Blood* 92 (1998): 1549–1555.

Rosenberg, S.A. "Karnofsky Memorial Lecture—The Immunotherapy and Gene Therapy of Cancer." *J Clin Oncol* 10 (1992): 180–199.

Rosenberg, S.A. (ed.). *Principles and Practice of the Biologic Therapy of Cancer,* 3rd ed. Philadelphia: Lippincott, Williams and Wilkins, (2000)

Rosenberg, S.A., J.C. Yang, and N.P. Restifo. "Cancer Immunotherapy—Moving Beyond Current Vaccines." *Nature Med* 10:9 (2004): 909–915.

Slavin, S., A. Nagler, E. Naparstek, et al. "Nonmyeloablative Stem Cell Transplantation and Cell Therapy as an Alternative to Conventional Bone Marrow Transplantation with Lethal Cytoreduction for the Treatment of Malignant and Nonmalignant Hematologic diseases." *Blood* 91 (1998): 756–763.

Vermorken, J.B., et al: "Active Specific Immunotherapy for Stage II and Stage III Human Colon Cancer: A Randomised Trial." *Lancet* 353 (1999): 345–350.

von Eschenbach, A.C. "A Vision for the National Cancer Program in the United States." *Nature Rev Cancer* 4:10 (2004).

Waldmann, Herman. "A Personal History of the CAMPATH-1H Antibody." *Med Oncol* 19:Suppl (2002): S3–S9.

Wood, Gary. *J Neuro-Oncol* 8:2 (2000).

Chapter 10: Winter Worm, Summer Grass

Halpern, G.M. *Cordyceps: China's Healing Mushroom.* New York: Avery Publishing, 1998.

Halpern, G.M. *Healing Mushrooms.* Garden City Park, NY: Square One, 2007.

Holliday, J.C., et al. "Analysis of Quality and Techniques for Hybridization of Medicinal Fungus *Cordyceps sinensis* (Berk.) Sacc. (Ascomycetes)." *Int J Medic Mushr* 6:2 (2004): 151–164.

Hsu, T.H., et al. "A Comparison of the Chemical Composition and Bioactive Ingredients of the Chinese Medicinal Mushroom DongChongXiaCao, Its Counterfeit and Mimic and Fermented Mycelium of *Cordyceps sinensis.*" *Food Chem* 78:4 (2002): 463–469.

Jones, K. "The Potential Health Benefits of Purple Corn." *HerbalGram* 85 (2005): 46–49.

Kiho, T., et al. "Structural Features and Hypoglycemic Activity of a Polysaccharide (CS-F10) from the Cultured Mycelium of *Cordyceps sinensis.*" *Biol Pharm Bull* 22 (1999): 966–970.

Pegler, D.N., et al. "The Chinese Caterpillar Fungus." *Mycologist* 8 (1994): 3–5.

Pereira, J. "Summer-plant-winter-worm." *NY J Med* 1 (1843): 128–132.

Siu, K.M., et al. "Pharmacological Basis of 'Yin-nourishing' and 'Yang-invigorating' Actions of *Cordyceps,* a Chinese Tonic Herb." *Life Sci* 76:4 (2004): 385–395.

Steinkraus, D.C., et al. "Chinese Caterpillar Fungus and World Record Runners." *Am Entomol* Winter (1994): 235–239.

Wang, Q., et al. "Comparison of Some Pharmacological Effects Between *Cordyceps sinensis* and *Cephalosporium sinensis.*" *Bull Chin Materia Med* 12 (1987): 682–684.

Yamaguchi, N., et al. "Augmentation of Various Immune Reactivities of Tumor-bearing Hosts with an Extract of *Cordyceps sinensis.*" *Biotherapy* 2:3 (1990): 199–205.

Zhang, C.K., et al. "Nourishment of *Cordyceps sinensis* Mycelium." *Weishengwuxue Tongbao* 19:3 (1992): 129–133.

Zhang, M., et al. "Notes on the Alpine *Cordyceps* of China and Nearby Nations." *Mycotaxon* 66 (1998): 215–229.

Zhang, Z., et al. "Clinical and Laboratory Studies of Jinshuibao in Scavenging Oxygen Free Radicals in Elderly Senescent Xuzheng Patients." *J Admin Trad Chin Med* 5 (1995): 14–18.

Zhu, J.S., G.M. Halpern, K. Jones. "The Scientific Rediscovery of an Ancient Chinese Herbal Medicine: *Cordyceps sinensis.*" *J Altern Complement Med* 3 (1998): 239–303.

Chapter 11: The Quest for Common Ground

Dawkins, Richard. *River Out of Eden.* London: Weidenfeld & Nicholson, 1995.

Diamond, Jared. *The Third Chimpanzee.* New York: Harper Collins, 1992.

Feyerabend, Paul. "How to Defend Society Against Science." In Klemke, E.D., R. Hollinger, and DW Rudge. *Philosophy of Science.* New York: Prometheus Books, 1998.

Feyerabend, Paul. *Against Method.* London: Verso, 1993.

Foucault, Michel. *Madness and Civilization.* New York: Vintage Books, 1988.

Illich, I. *Limits to Medicine.* London: Marion Boyars, 2002.

Kuhn, T. "Objectivity, Value Judgment and Theory Choice." In Klemke, E.D., R. Hollinger, and D.W. Rudge (eds.). *Philosophy of Science.* New York: Prometheus Books, 1998.

Laing, R.D. *Politics of Experience.* London: Penguin Books, 1967.

MacIntyre, Alasdair. *Whose Justice? Which Rationality?* London: Duckworth, 1998.

Monod, Jacques. *Chance and Necessity.* New York: Alfred A. Knopf, 1971.

Stamets, P. *Mycelium Running: How Mushrooms Can Save the World.* Berkeley, CA: Ten Speed Press, 2005.

Szasz, Thomas. *Ideology and Insanity.* London: Calder and Boyars, 1973.

Wilson, Edward O. *Consilience.* London: Little Brown, 1998.

Index